BOHO
BRAIDS

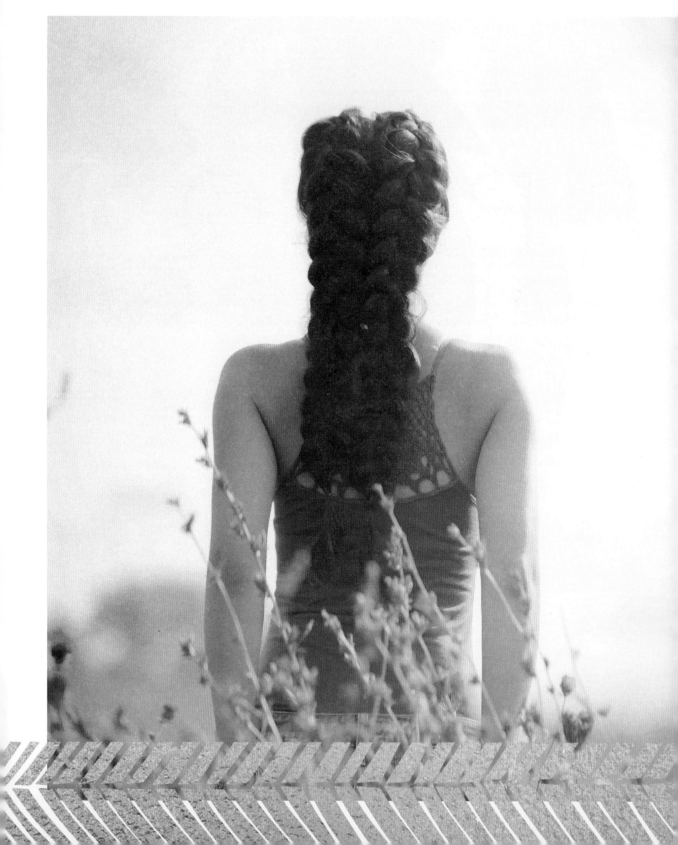

BOHO BRAIDS

40 modern, free-spirited hairstyles

By Heidi Marie Garrett & Katie Rossi

CONTENTS

Hair Basics 11

Basic Braid. 12

Fishtail Braid 13

French Braid. 14

Dutch Braid. 16

Pancaking. 18

Basic Bun 20

Style Prep. 21

Beach Waves. 22

Teasing. .24

A Better Ponytail Elastic. 25

Attaching Clip-In Extensions. 26

Finishing Your Style 28

Accessorizing 29

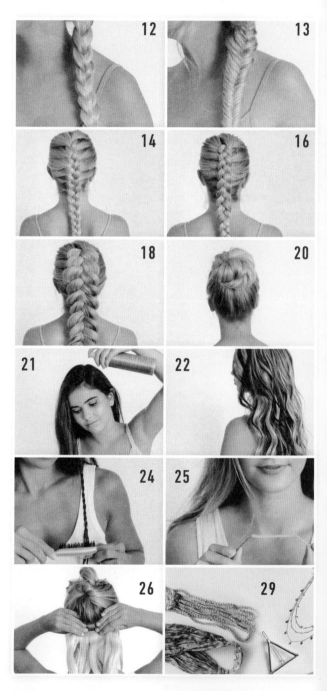

The Styles. 31

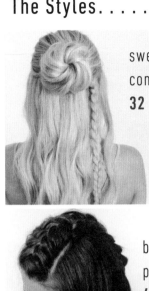

sweet
confection
32

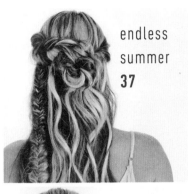

endless
summer
37

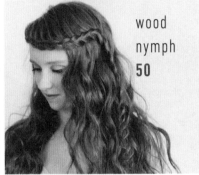

california
vibes
40

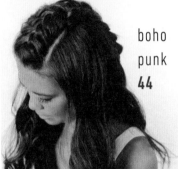

boho
punk
44

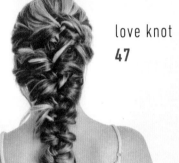

love knot
47

wood
nymph
50

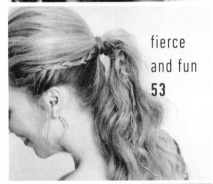

fierce
and fun
53

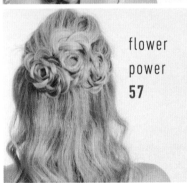

flower
power
57

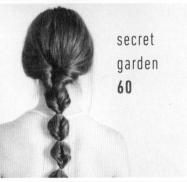

secret
garden
60

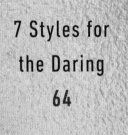

7 Styles for
the Daring
64

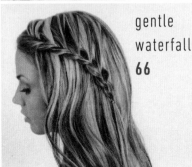

gentle
waterfall
66

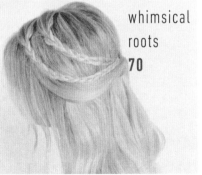

whimsical
roots
70

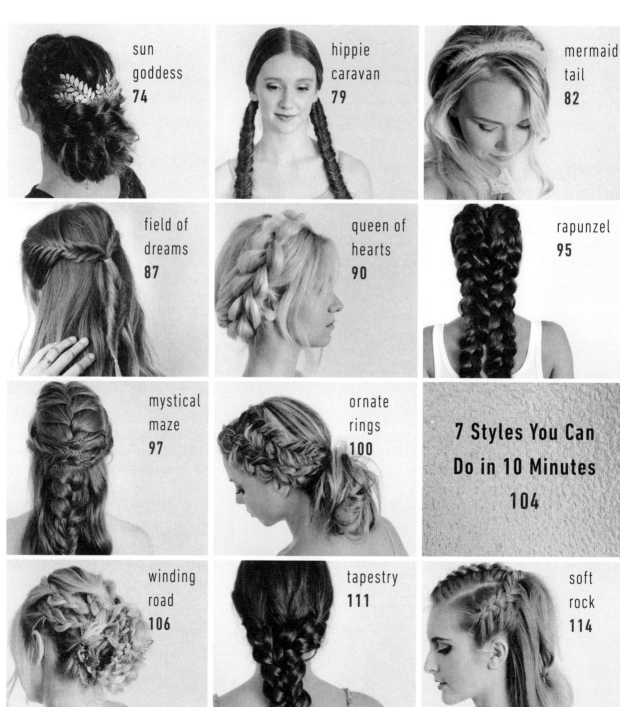

sun
goddess
74

hippie
caravan
79

mermaid
tail
82

field of
dreams
87

queen of
hearts
90

rapunzel
95

mystical
maze
97

ornate
rings
100

**7 Styles You Can
Do in 10 Minutes
104**

winding
road
106

tapestry
111

soft
rock
114

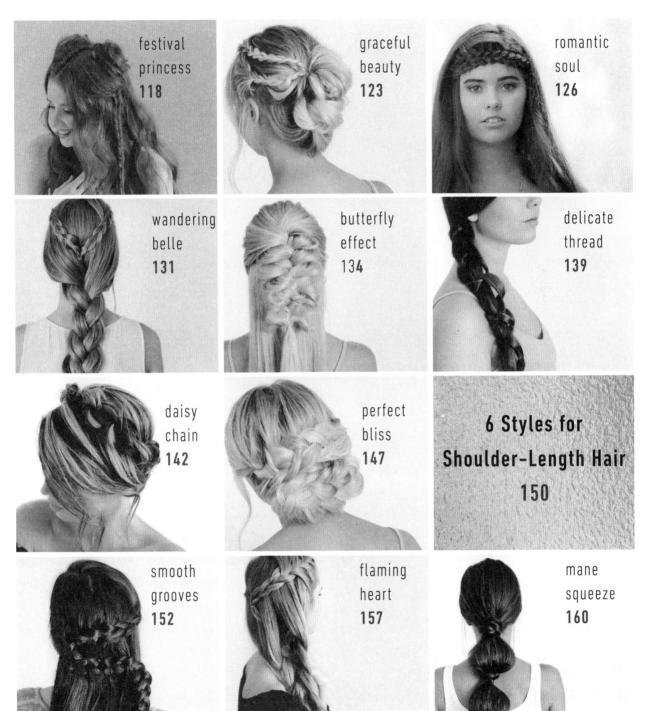

festival princess 118

graceful beauty 123

romantic soul 126

wandering belle 131

butterfly effect 134

delicate thread 139

daisy chain 142

perfect bliss 147

6 Styles for Shoulder-Length Hair 150

smooth grooves 152

flaming heart 157

mane squeeze 160

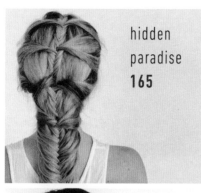

hidden
paradise
165

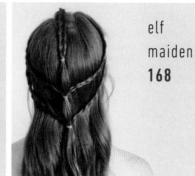

elf
maiden
168

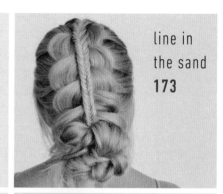

line in
the sand
173

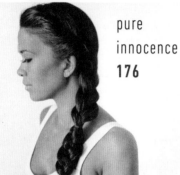

pure
innocence
176

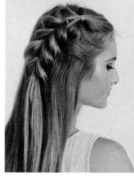

boho
ingénue
178

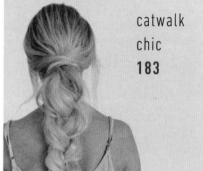

catwalk
chic
183

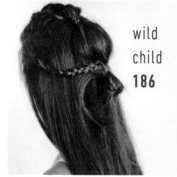

wild
child
186

About the Authors 190
Acknowledgments 191

INTRODUCTION

The modern bohemian girl takes on the essence of a hippie, yet remains grounded in her pursuit of modern ideas and style. She enjoys experimenting with music, fashion, and art, and has a wild imagination that gives her the confidence to stand out from the crowd. The boho girl congregates with her like-minded friends at music festivals and gatherings that celebrate self-expression, freedom, friendship, and love.

Because she isn't afraid to try unique things, the boho girl loves unconventional hairstyles that feel effortless—which is why she loves messy, unstructured braids. She wears transitional styles that last for multiple days, giving the impression that her hair was last touched by a pillowcase rather than a brush.

Are you ready to embrace your inner boho girl? Tap into your creative side with the various styles in this book. Make them as loose and textured as you can—these braids are meant to be unpolished in the best way possible!

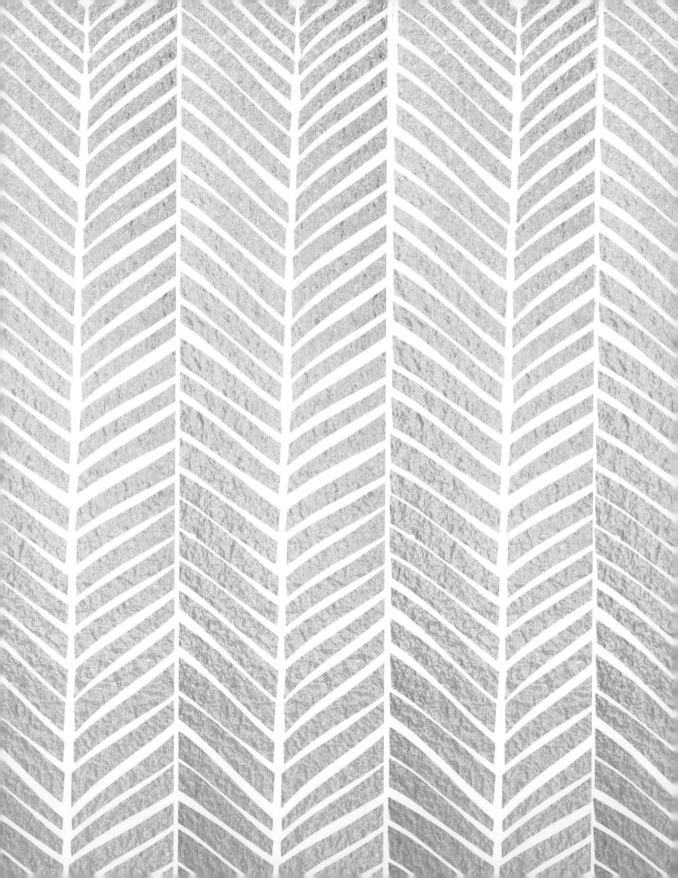

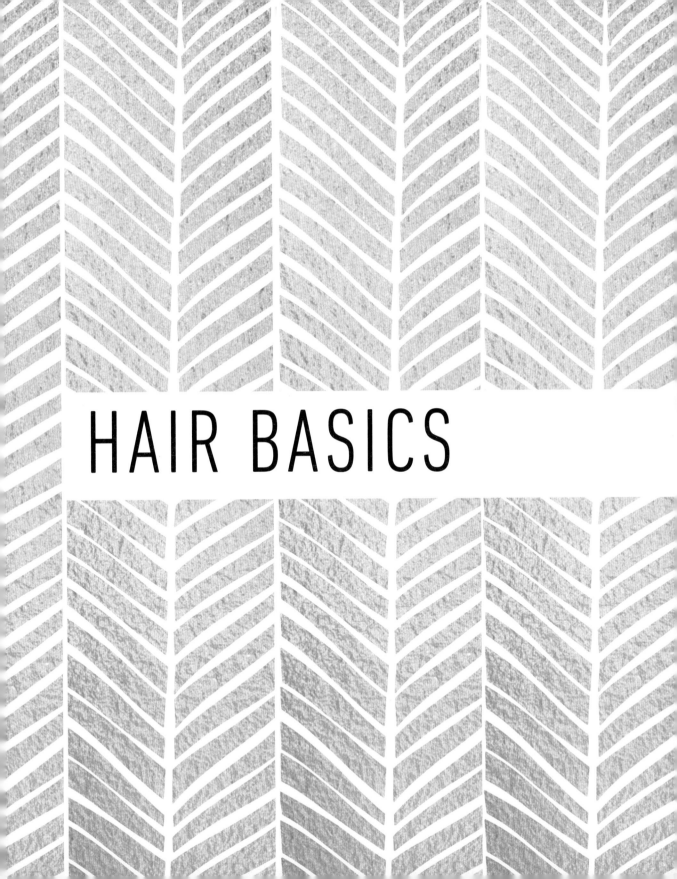

HAIR BASICS

BASIC BRAID

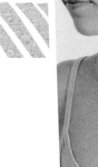

Learning how to do a basic three-strand braid gives you the foundation from which you can create other, more complicated braids.

1 After gathering the desired amount of hair for your braid, split your hair into three equal sections.

2 Cross the right section over the middle section, sliding the middle section off to the right as you do so.

3 Cross the left section over the middle section, sliding the middle section off to the left as you do so.

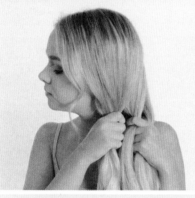

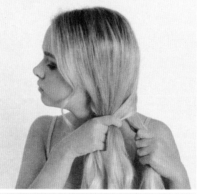

4 Cross the right section over the middle section, sliding the middle section off to the right as you do so.

5 Cross the left section over the middle section, sliding the middle section off to the left as you do.

6 Repeat steps 2 through 5 until you reach the end of your hair.

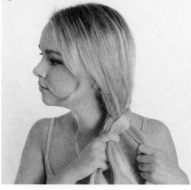

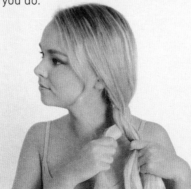

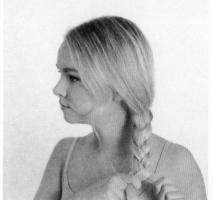

FISHTAIL BRAID

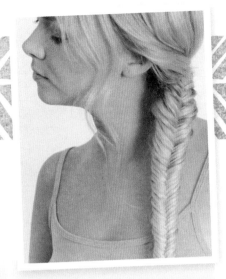

A fishtail braid is beautifully unique but requires a bit of patience. To make the fishtail pattern obvious, work with only tiny strands of hair.

1 Split your hair into two equal sections.

2 Using the index finger of your right hand, separate a tiny strand of hair from the outside of the right section.

3 Cross the tiny strand over to the section on the left side and join them.

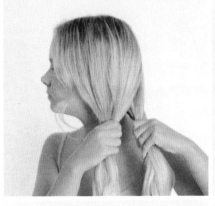

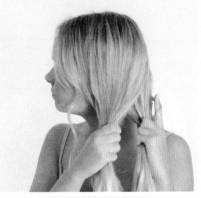

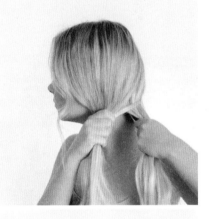

4 Using the index finger of your left hand, separate a tiny strand of hair from the outside of the left section.

5 Cross the tiny strand all the way over to the right side and join them.

6 Repeat steps 2 through 5 until you reach the end of your hair.

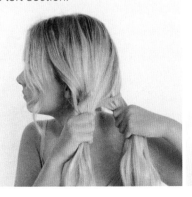

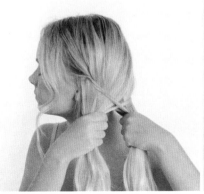

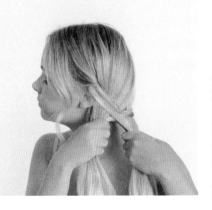

FRENCH BRAID

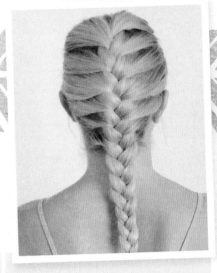

A French braid incorporates the simple techniques and principles of the basic braid, but involves adding in hair as you create it.

1 After choosing where you want to start the braid, take a section of hair and separate it into three smaller sections.

2 Begin creating a basic braid by crossing the right section over the middle section, sliding the middle section off to the right as you do so.

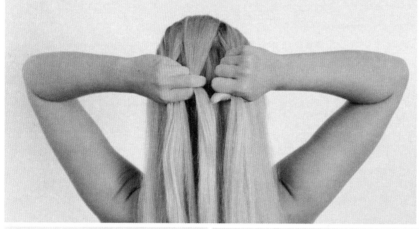

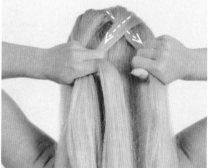

3 Cross the left section over the middle section, sliding the middle section off to the left as you do so.

4 Holding the braid in your left hand, place each section between your fingers. Use your right hand to section off a sliver of hair on the right side next to the braid.

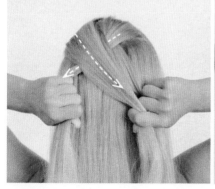

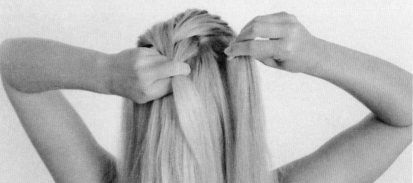

5 Add the sliver of hair to the right section. Cross this section over the middle.

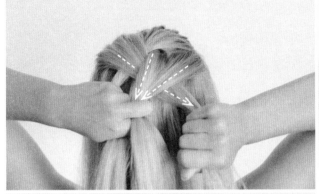

6 While holding the braid in your right hand, use your left hand to section off a sliver of hair on the left side next to the braid.

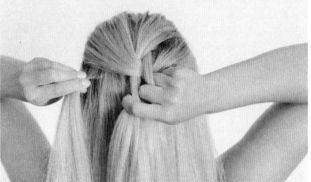

7 Add the sliver of hair to the left section. Cross this section over the middle.

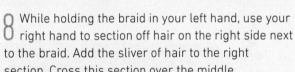
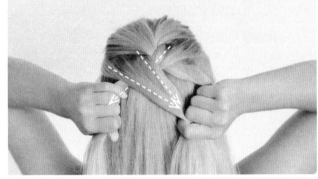

8 While holding the braid in your left hand, use your right hand to section off hair on the right side next to the braid. Add the sliver of hair to the right section. Cross this section over the middle.

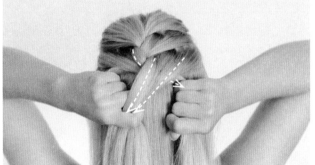

9 While holding the braid in your right hand, use your left hand to section off a sliver of hair on the left side next to the braid. Add the sliver of hair to the left section. Cross this section over the middle.

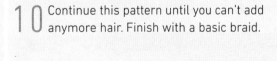
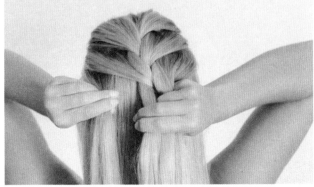

10 Continue this pattern until you can't add anymore hair. Finish with a basic braid.

DUTCH BRAID

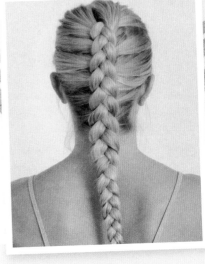

The Dutch braid is essentially an inside-out version of the French braid, with the middle section crossing up and over the side sections.

1 After choosing where you want to start the braid, take a larger section of hair and separate it into three smaller sections.

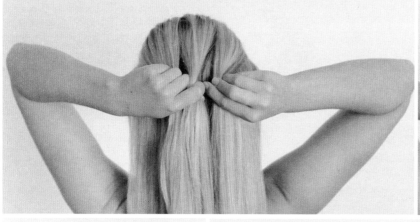

2 Cross the middle section over the right section, sliding the right section under to the middle as you do so.

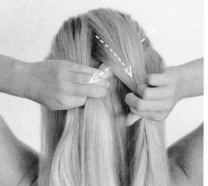

3 Cross the middle section over the left section, sliding the left section under the middle as you do so.

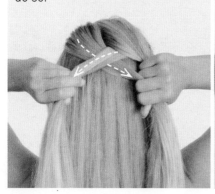

4 Holding the braid in your left hand (see "French Braid" step 4 for reference), use your right hand to section off hair on the right side next to the braid.

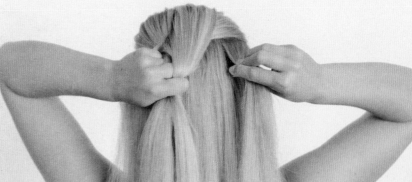

5 Add the sliver of hair to the right section. Cross the middle section over the right side section.

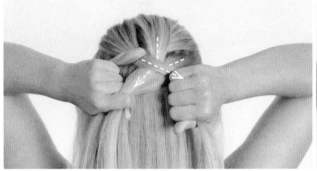

6 While holding the braid in your right hand, use your left hand to section off hair on the left side next to the braid. Add the sliver of hair to the left section. Cross the middle section over the left side section.

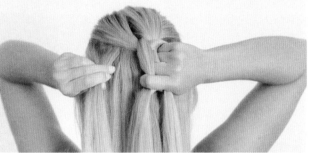

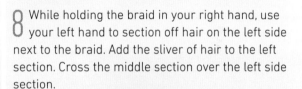

7 While holding the braid in your left hand, use your right hand to section off hair on the right side next to the braid. Add the sliver of hair to the right section. Cross the middle section over the right side section.

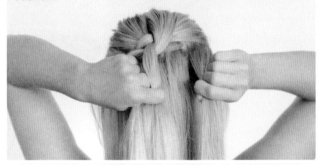

8 While holding the braid in your right hand, use your left hand to section off hair on the left side next to the braid. Add the sliver of hair to the left section. Cross the middle section over the left side section.

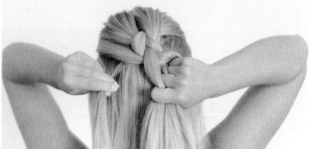

9 Continue this pattern until you can't add anymore hair. Finish with a basic braid.

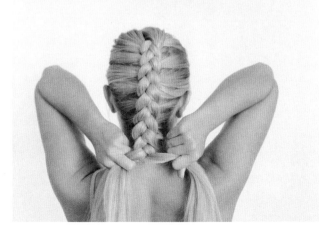

As you learn to Dutch braid, take it slow. It's easy to accidentally revert to doing a French braid while you're in the middle of creating your Dutch braid.

PANCAKING

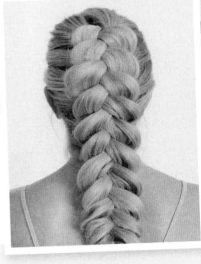

Pancaking is a technique that allows you to make your braids appear fuller and chunkier by simply pulling on the loops of the braid.

1 Starting at the loops near the elastic band, gently pull each loop while holding the elastic band with your opposite hand.

2 Moving up the braid to the next set of loops, gently pull each loop.

3 Continue moving up the braid loop by loop until you've loosened the braid to the desired fullness.

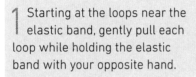

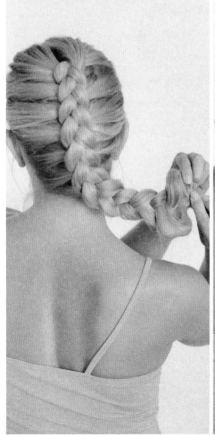

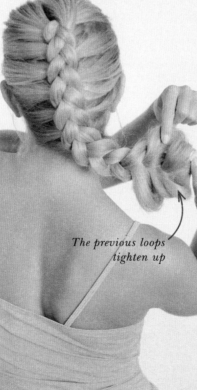

The previous loops tighten up

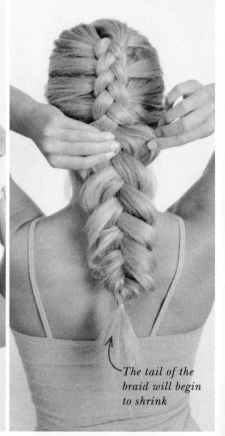

The tail of the braid will begin to shrink

Dutch braid

The Dutch braid is the easiest braid to pancake, because the loops are easy to see and grab onto.

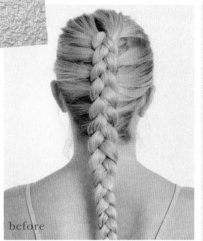

before

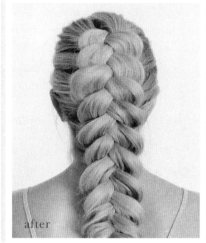

after

French braid

When pancaking a French braid, concentrate mostly on the basic braid at the bottom. However, you should also gently loosen the main braid.

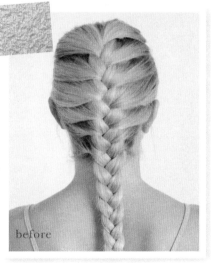

before

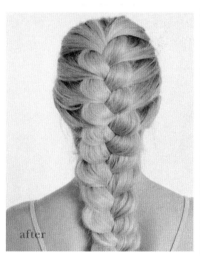

after

Fishtail braid

Don't be afraid to get extra aggressive when pancaking a fishtail braid. This braid is meant to be textured and messy.

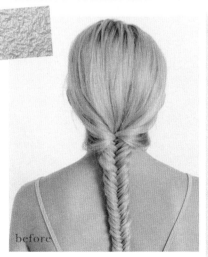

before

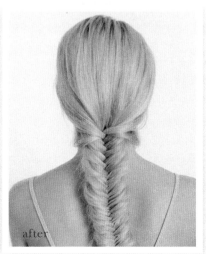

after

BASIC BUN

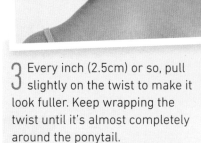

Many of the styles in this book incorporate a loose, messy bun into the braided looks. The following is the trick to achieving this type of bun.

1 Place your hair into a ponytail. Loosely twist the ponytail to the right.

2 Begin wrapping the twist loosely in a clockwise direction around the ponytail holder.

3 Every inch (2.5cm) or so, pull slightly on the twist to make it look fuller. Keep wrapping the twist until it's almost completely around the ponytail.

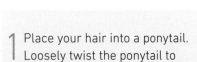

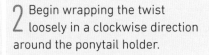

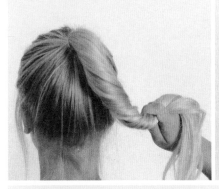

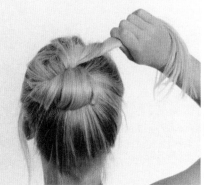

4 Slide in bobby pins from the outer perimeter toward the center of the bun. Evenly space the pins so they create an asterisk shape.

Don't open the bobby pins

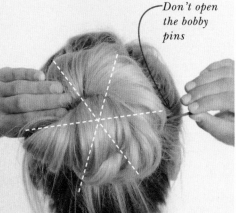

5 Loosen areas of the bun that appear to be tight. Add more bobby pins to secure any pieces that are too loose.

The bobby pins should be invisible

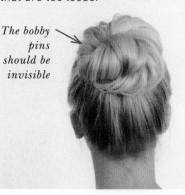

STYLE PREP

Prepping your hair and having the right supplies ready to use are just as important as the actual hairstyle itself. Start your braiding off right!

Applying Dry Shampoo

Dry shampoo is a wonderful way to extend the time in between washing your hair. It also provides texture for silkier hair types.

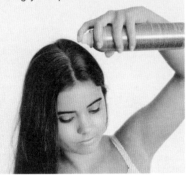

1 Holding the can 6 inches (15.25cm) from your scalp, spray a coat of dry shampoo along your part line.

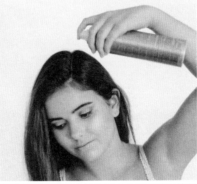

2 Take sections parallel to your original part and spray dry shampoo onto the part lines.

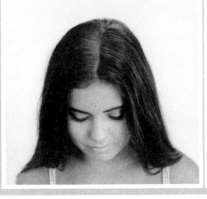

3 After spraying all of the sections, let the product dry completely and turn white.

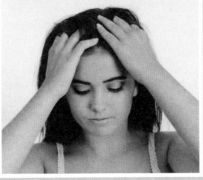

4 Place your fingers throughout the areas where you sprayed and rub in the product thoroughly.

SUPPLIES

Bobby pins

Make sure you have plenty of bobby pins out and ready before you start styling your hair.

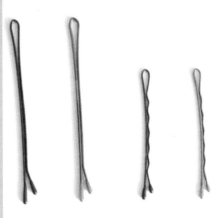

Elastic bands

Use small elastics instead of larger, bulkier ponytail holders to secure your braids.

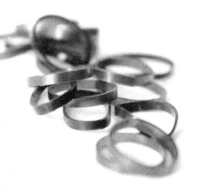

BEACH WAVES

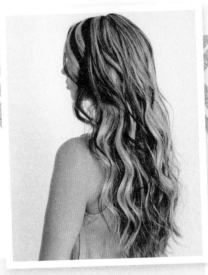

Due to their undone and textured appearance, beach waves are the perfect addition to any boho style. You can even style your hair the night before and wake up with natural-looking waves.

1 Start with perfectly dry hair. Section out the bottom portion and clip away the rest of your hair on top.

2 Take a small section from the bottom. Carefully wrap it in a spiraling manner around the barrel of the wand (from roots to tips). Keep it there for 10 seconds, and then release.

Point the wand downward toward the floor

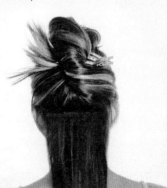

Leave the ends out to keep them straight

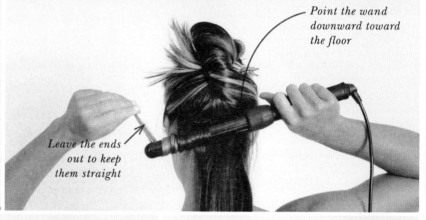

3 Wrap another section around the curling wand in the opposite direction of the previous wave. Keep it there for 10 seconds, and then release.

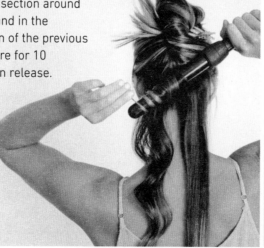

4 Repeat steps 2 and 3 until the bottom portion is done.

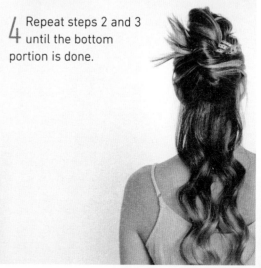

TOOLS

Curling wand or iron

Your curling wand should be the same circumference from the base to the tip.

Spray wax

This adds texture and shine to your beach waves.

Hair clips

Use these to clip your hair out of the way as you're working on other sections.

If your hair doesn't hold curl well, use a medium-barrel (1-inch; 25mm) curling wand. For looser waves—and if your hair holds curl well—use a large-barrel (1½-inch; 35mm) curling wand.

5 Section off another layer of hair and clip away the rest of your hair on top. Repeat steps 2 and 3 until this section is done.

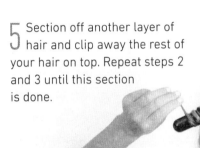

6 Keep moving up your head, sectioning and wrapping, until you've curled all of your hair.

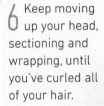
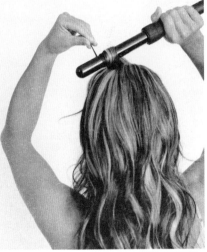

7 Flip your hair to each side and apply an even coat of spray wax to all of your hair.

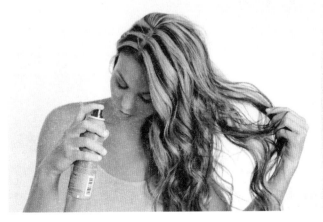

8 Flip your head upright and shake out your waves using your hands.

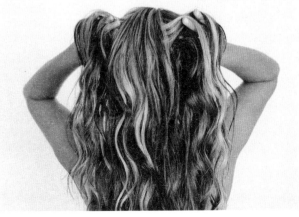

TEASING

To better play up your boho look, you can use these teasing techniques to give your finished style more texture and volume.

Basic teasing at the crown

1 Using ¾-inch (2cm) horizontal sections of hair, place the teeth of the teasing brush 2 inches (5cm) from your scalp.

2 Push the hair down toward the scalp. Bring the brush back up, and then push it down again. Repeat this process two to three times.

3 Continue taking horizontal sections and repeating this process until you've completed the crown area.

Teasing your beach waves

Take a medium-size section of hair and hold the bottom with your nondominant hand. Using the teeth of the brush, gently push the hairs at the curves of each wave up 1 inch (2.5cm). Repeat this process throughout your hair.

TOOLS

Teasing brush

A teasing brush should have firm bristles of different heights, and the head of the brush should be long and skinny.

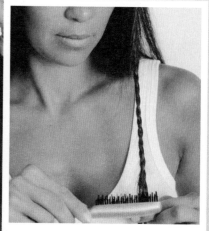

Teasing the end of your braid

Instead of using an elastic, you can tease your hair to secure your braid. Simply tangle the hair together by using the teeth of a brush, and then make small tapping motions in an upward direction at the end of the braid. Spritz it lightly with hairspray to finish.

A BETTER PONYTAIL ELASTIC

Do you have trouble maintaining your hair in a ponytail? This simple step-by-step shows you how to create one with true staying power.

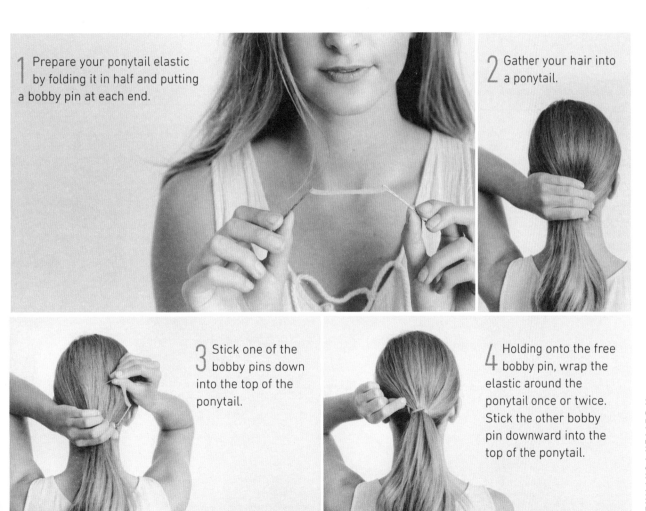

1 Prepare your ponytail elastic by folding it in half and putting a bobby pin at each end.

2 Gather your hair into a ponytail.

3 Stick one of the bobby pins down into the top of the ponytail.

4 Holding onto the free bobby pin, wrap the elastic around the ponytail once or twice. Stick the other bobby pin downward into the top of the ponytail.

ATTACHING CLIP-IN EXTENSIONS

Adding clip-in hair extensions can instantly upgrade your hairstyle. They can be used to not only make your overall hair fuller and longer, but they can also be incorporated into your braids and updos.

TOOLS

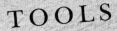

Hair extensions

Clip-in hair extensions come in various lengths, colors, and thicknesses. Each pack of hair will generally include different-size wefts ranging from one clip to four clips across.

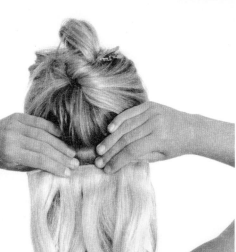

1 Make a horizontal part. Clip away the hair above the part.

2 Tease small sections near your scalp where the extension clips will attach.

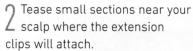
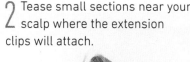
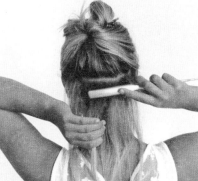

3 Spray each of the teased areas with hairspray.

4 Hook the clips onto each teased section and snap them shut. Repeat this process for each section.

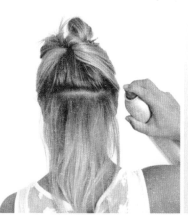

HAIR BASICS

26

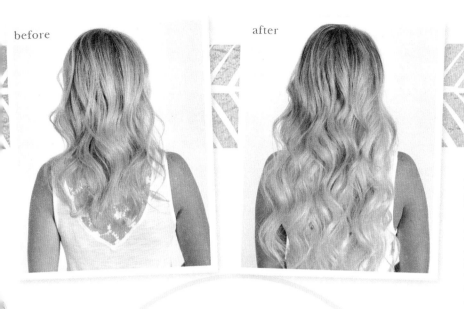

before

after

Do your research before investing in clip-in hair extensions; they should last you years if they are properly taken care of. Don't go for cheap hair extensions, as they tend to tangle more easily and look stringy.

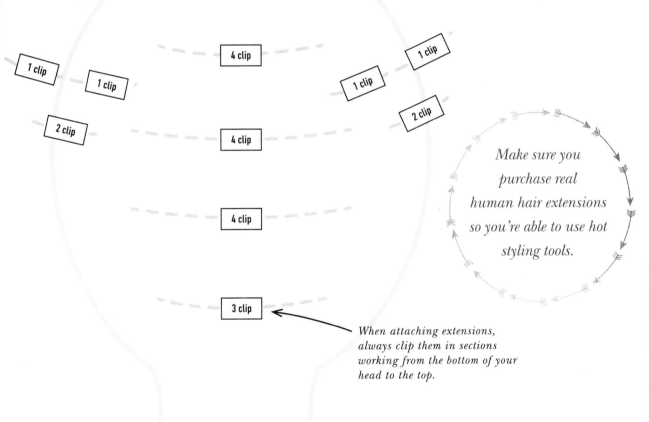

1 clip

1 clip

2 clip

4 clip

4 clip

4 clip

3 clip

1 clip

1 clip

2 clip

Make sure you purchase real human hair extensions so you're able to use hot styling tools.

When attaching extensions, always clip them in sections working from the bottom of your head to the top.

FINISHING YOUR STYLE

In order for your hairstyle to last all day, it's important to know how to use bobby pins, as well as hairspray and spray wax, to complete your style.

Hairspray vs. Spray wax

The difference between hairspray and spray wax comes down to their individual purpose. Hairspray is more commonly used to help hold the style in place, whereas spray wax is used to add texture to the hair while still allowing movement. Spray wax should be worked through the hair after application; however, hairspray simply needs to dry after spraying.

Both products should be held about 8 inches (20cm) from your head when spraying. Try not to excessively spray the product, because your hair will end up feeling stiff, oily, or heavy. For safety reasons, read the directions on the product labels before using them.

Bobby pins

Bobby pins vary in size, color, and strength. Large roller pins are great for heavy or thick hair, and also help secure larger buns. Regular-size bobby pins are multipurpose and work for all hair types.

Keep bobby pins closed when sliding them into your hair. This allows just the right amount of hair to wedge between the sides of the pin. If you open it before you slide it in, you risk grabbing too much hair, which doesn't allow the pin to do its job.

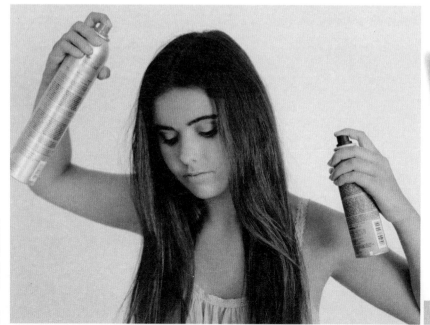

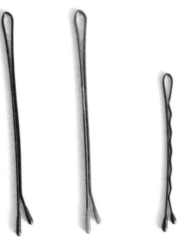

ACCESSORIZING

Personalize your boho hairstyle by experimenting with different hair accessories. Whether you like to mix and match, layer your accessories, or keep things simple, you'll be the center of attention when you adorn your hair with one of these.

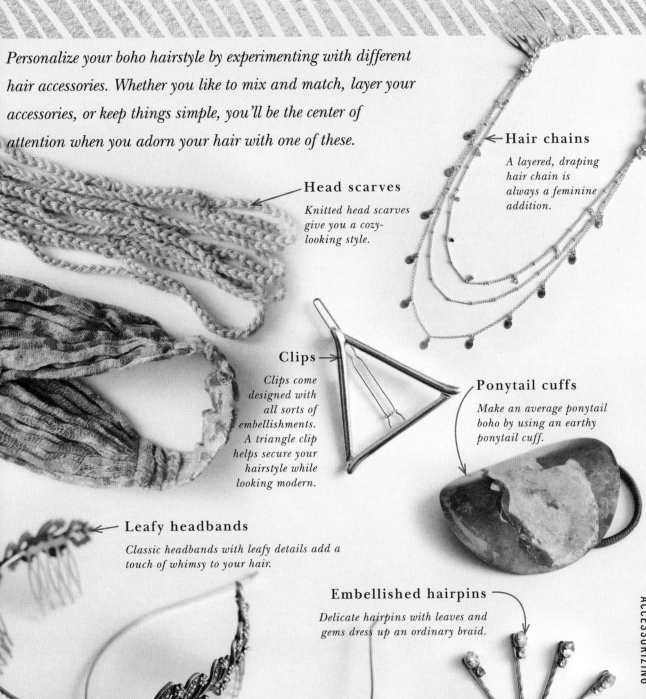

Hair chains

A layered, draping hair chain is always a feminine addition.

Head scarves

Knitted head scarves give you a cozy-looking style.

Clips

Clips come designed with all sorts of embellishments. A triangle clip helps secure your hairstyle while looking modern.

Ponytail cuffs

Make an average ponytail boho by using an earthy ponytail cuff.

Leafy headbands

Classic headbands with leafy details add a touch of whimsy to your hair.

Embellished hairpins

Delicate hairpins with leaves and gems dress up an ordinary braid.

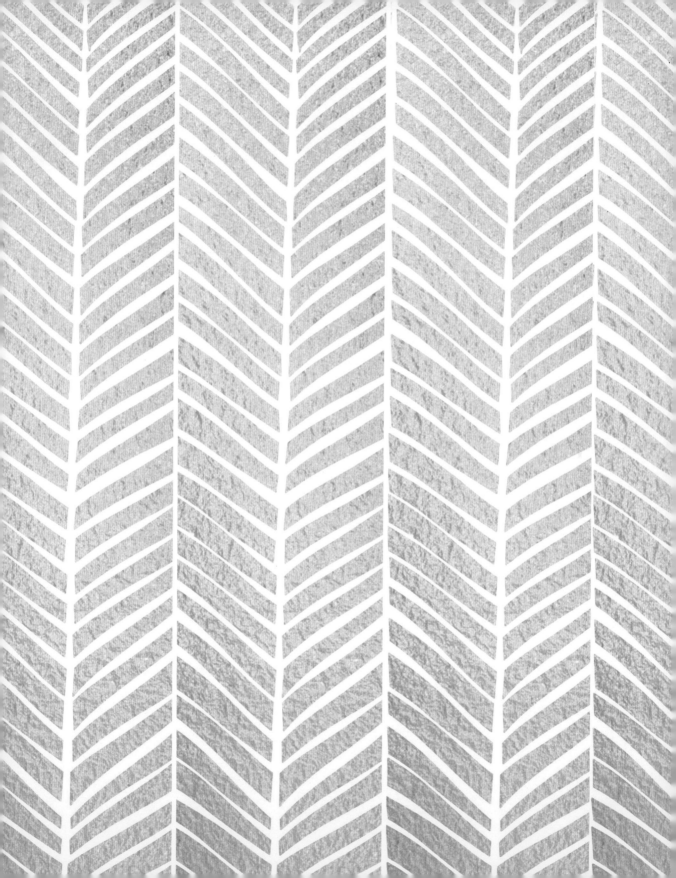

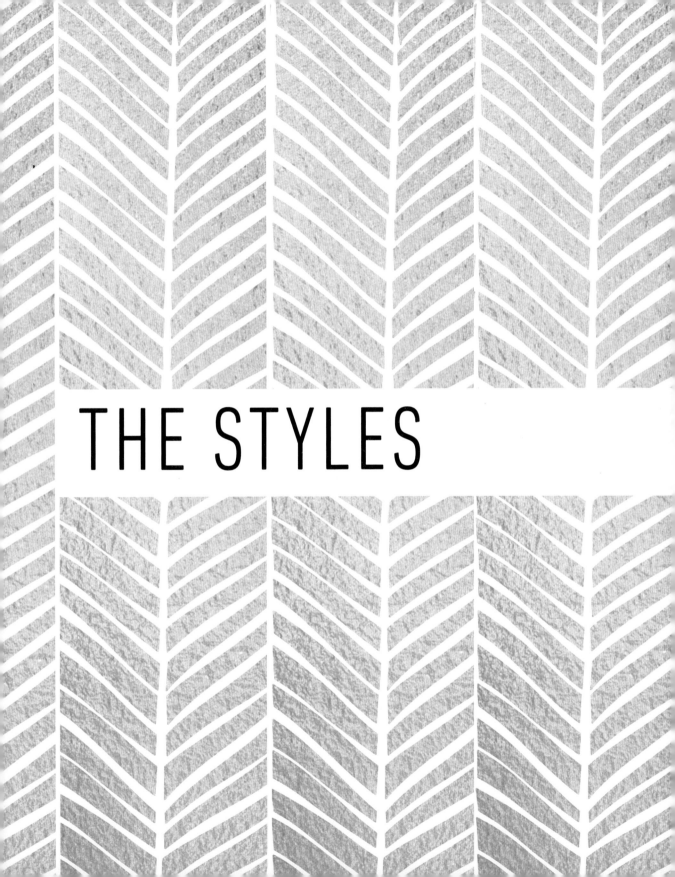

THE STYLES

sweet
CONFECTION

*This style, with its **loose bun** and **textured braid,** is incredibly versatile. It's sophisticated enough to wear in an office setting, yet playful enough for a trip to the nearest sweet shop. No matter what you do, you'll be looking your best!*

difficulty
easy

minimum hair length
top of shoulders

what you'll need
large-barrel (1½ in.; 35mm) curling wand or iron

hair clip

clear ponytail elastic (or a color that matches your hair)

bobby pins

hairspray

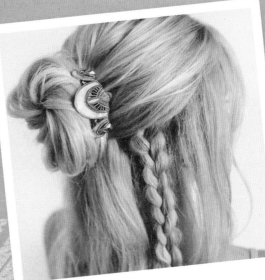

accessorize it!
Slide the comb of a bun pin into the side of the bun to add a dressier style element.

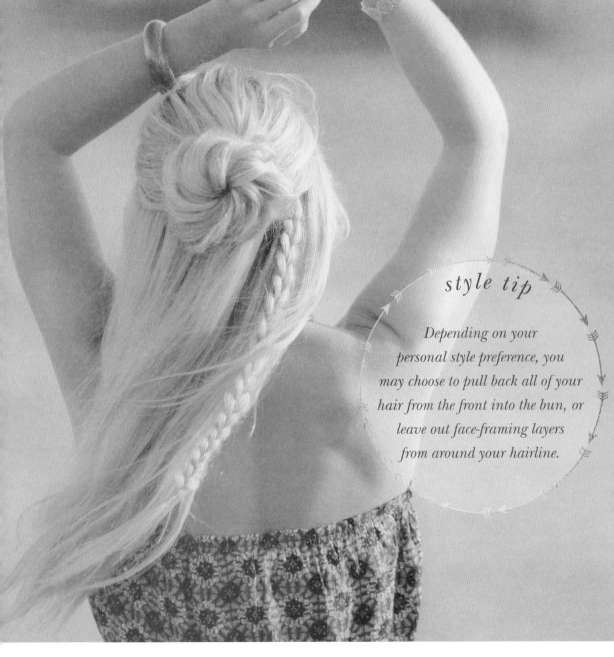

style tip

Depending on your
personal style preference, you
may choose to pull back all of your
hair from the front into the bun, or
leave out face-framing layers
from around your hairline.

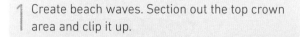

1 Create beach waves. Section out the top crown area and clip it up.

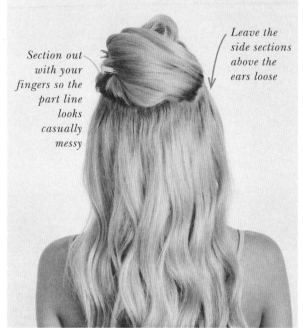

Section out with your fingers so the part line looks casually messy

Leave the side sections above the ears loose

2 Take a small- to medium-sized section of hair above and behind one ear and create a basic braid. Secure the end with an elastic.

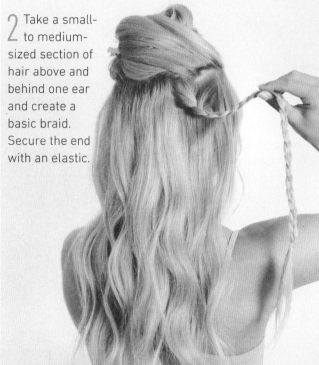

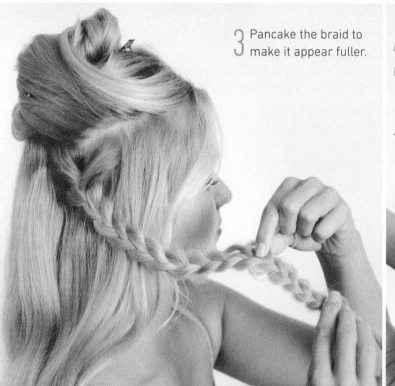

3 Pancake the braid to make it appear fuller.

4 Place all of the hair from the top section into a loose ponytail. Secure with an elastic.

Elastic band

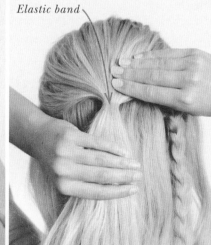

5 Loosely twist and wrap the ponytail to create a bun. Slide bobby pins into the center of the bun to secure it. Gently pull pieces of the bun and surrounding area of hair to create fullness and texture. Finish the style with hairspray.

Keep the bobby pins close to the scalp

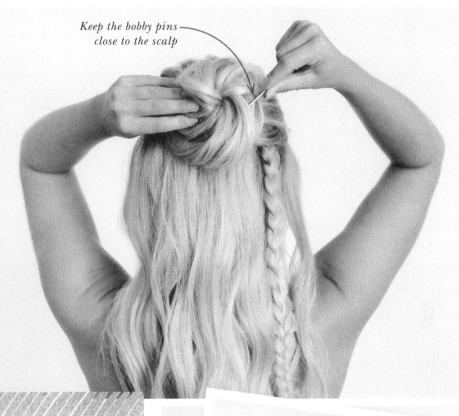

FINISHED LOOK

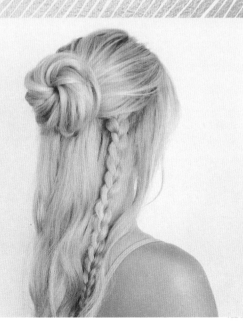

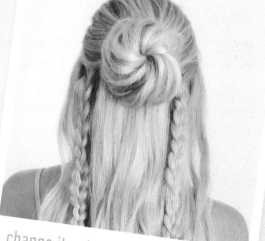

change it up!
Make a second braid next to the original braid.

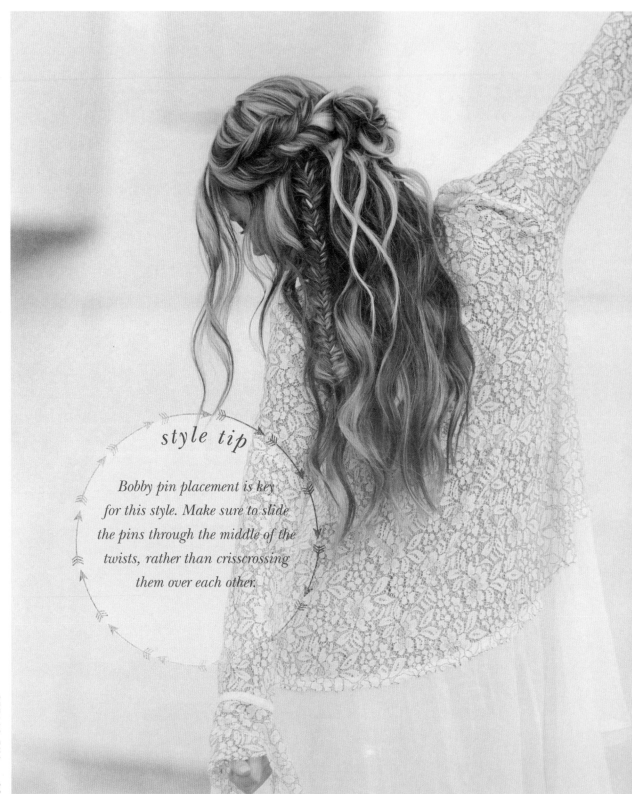

style tip

Bobby pin placement is key
for this style. Make sure to slide
the pins through the middle of the
twists, rather than crisscrossing
them over each other.

ENDLESS
summer

*Capture the feeling of a memorable, everlasting summer with this romantic style. With **pretty twists** and a **small yet loose fishtail,** it's perfect for everything from a day out at the pool to a bonfire party at night.*

difficulty
intermediate

minimum hair length
shoulder blades

what you'll need
large-barrel (1½ in.; 35mm) curling wand or iron
bobby pins
clear small elastics (or a color that matches your hair)
hairspray

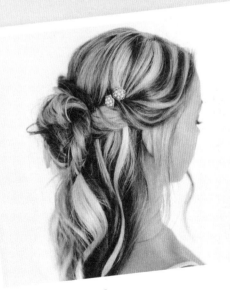

accessorize it!
For a simple yet sweet adornment, slide a couple delicate, decorative bobby pins above the single twist. This style already appears elaborate, so less is more.

1 Create beach waves. Take a section of hair from the heavier side of your part, leaving hair out above your ear. Loosely twist the section away from your face.

2 Secure with bobby pins in the middle of your head at the back.

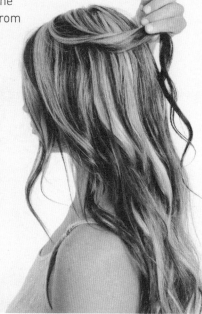

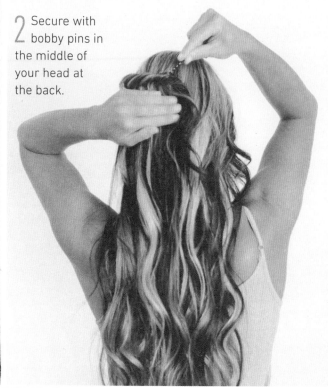

3 Take a section of hair below the previous twist, twist it toward your face, and lay it under the previous twist. Secure with bobby pins.

4 On the other side of your part, twist a section away from your face. Secure with bobby pins.

Keep the bobby pins close to the scalp

5 Using the sections hanging down from the back middle area, create a loose bun. Slide bobby pins into the center of the bun to secure it.

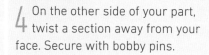

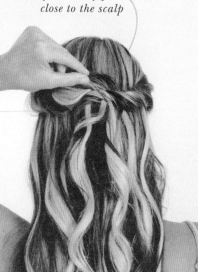

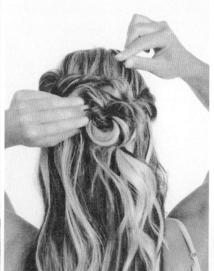

6 Take a small section of hair to the left of the bun and create a fishtail braid. Secure with an elastic.

7 Pancake the braid to make it appear fuller.

8 Loosen up the bun or any area that may be too tight. Finish the style with hairspray.

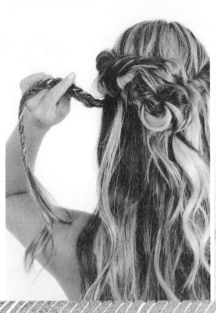 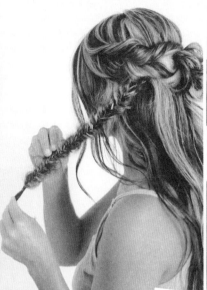 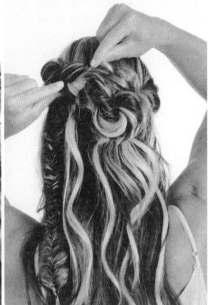

FINISHED LOOK

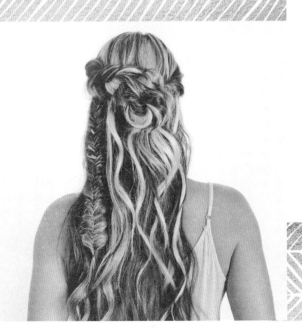

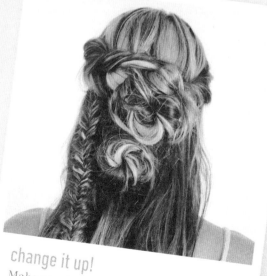

change it up!
Make another small bun below the first one.

CALIFORNIA
vibes

*This **messy, textured hairstyle** brings out the California girl in all of us. Perfect for hair that hasn't been freshly washed, simply spray on some dry shampoo and begin braiding. You can then head outdoors to bask in the sunshine.*

difficulty
intermediate

minimum hair length
shoulder blades

what you'll need
dry shampoo
comb
clear small elastics (or a color that matches your hair)
bobby pins
hairspray

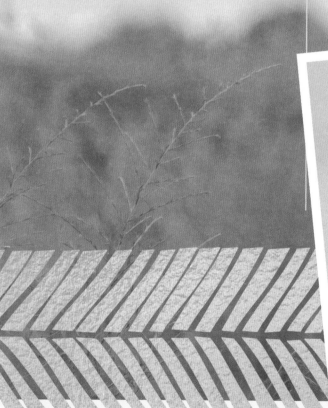

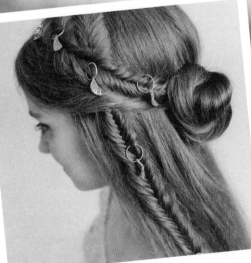

accessorize it!
Place some hair rings down one or two of the braids for some extra flair.

Wash your hair the night before and either use a hair dryer or allow to air-dry overnight. In the morning, spray a moderate amount of dry shampoo at the roots of your hair in 1-inch (2.5cm) sections, focusing mainly on the top and sides. Finally, use your fingers to "scrub" your scalp until the roots feel dry.

1 Prep your hair using dry shampoo. Part your hair deep to one side.

2 Working with the heavier side of the part, section out a piece of hair about 1 inch (2.5cm) wide going from your part down to your ear.

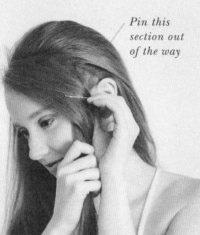

Pin this section out of the way

3 Make a Dutch fishtail braid behind the pinned section. Stop adding hair 3 inches (7.5cm) down. Finish braiding the remaining hair to the ends. Secure with an elastic.

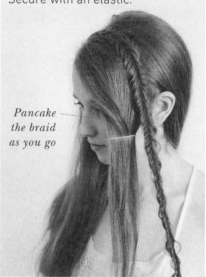

Pancake the braid as you go

4 Pin the braid out of the way. Start making a French fishtail braid right behind it, adding in random pieces from the frontmost section about 3 inches (7.5cm) down.

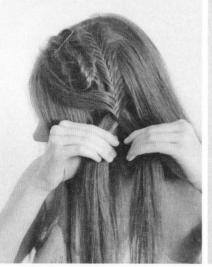

5 When the braid reaches the top of your ear, stop adding in hair. Keep braiding to the ends, pancaking as you go and secure with an elastic. Release the front braid from the bobby pin.

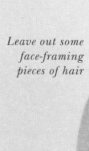

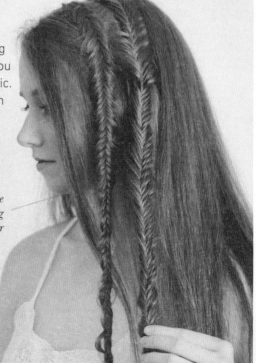

Leave out some face-framing pieces of hair

6 Unpin the 1-inch (2.5cm) section and twist it away from your face. Using crisscrossed bobby pins, pin it and the first braid together in back, slightly off-center.

7 On the other side of the part, gather a section of hair and pull it to the back of your head.

Include hair at the crown and any hair about 1 inch (2.5cm) above your ear

8 Loosely twist the section along with the bobby-pinned hair and form into a loose, messy bun. Secure the bun with pins. Finish the style with hairspray.

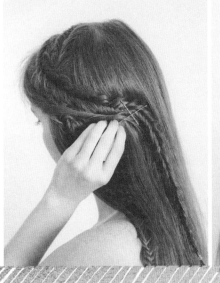

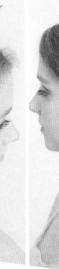

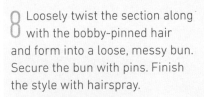

Place the bun over the criss-crossed bobby pins

FINISHED LOOK

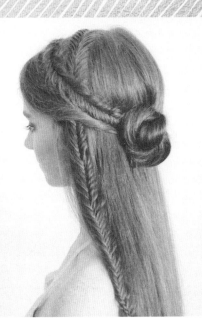

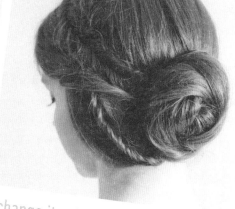

change it up!
Twist the remaining hair into a loose bun that wraps around the small bun.

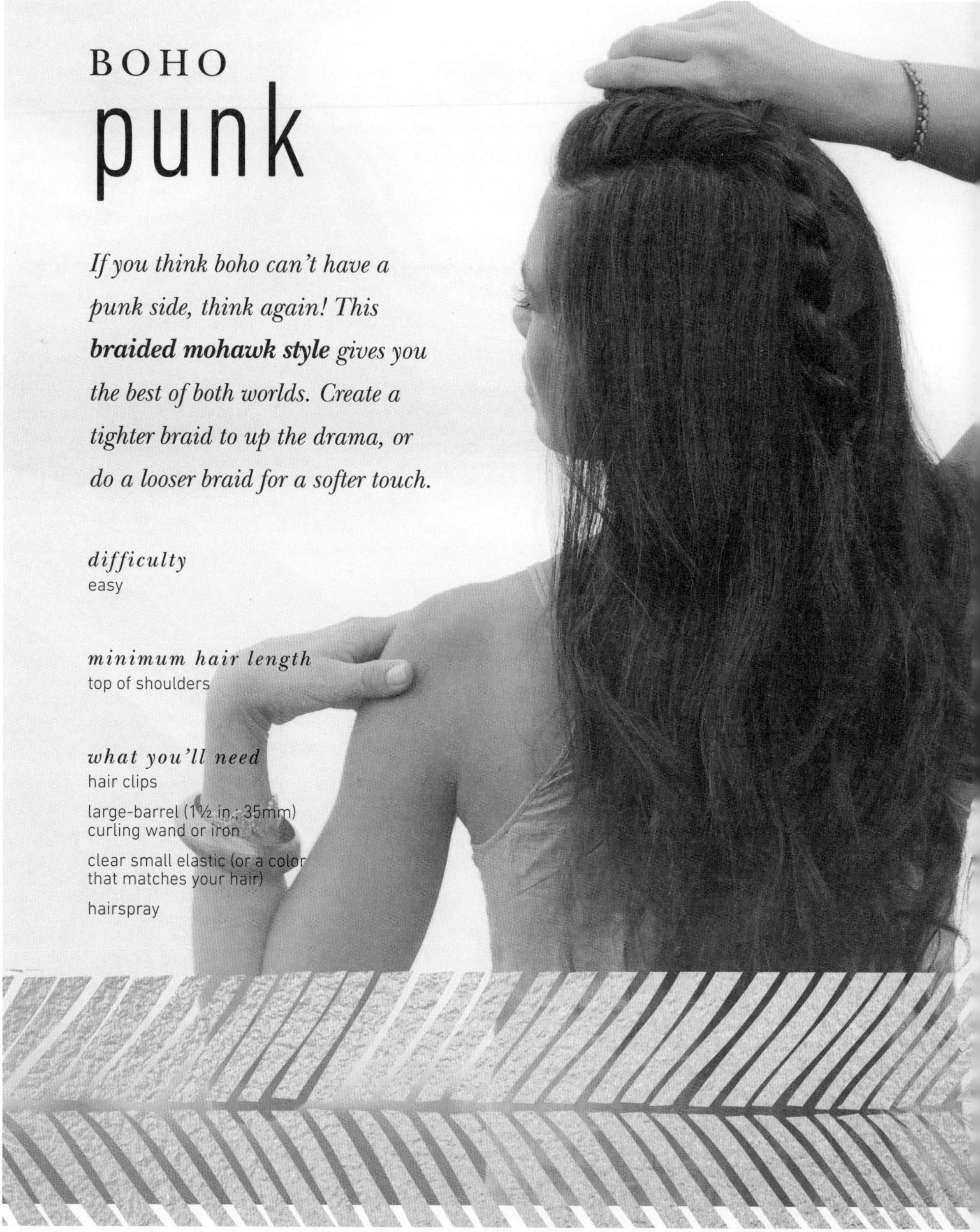

BOHO
punk

*If you think boho can't have a punk side, think again! This **braided mohawk style** gives you the best of both worlds. Create a tighter braid to up the drama, or do a looser braid for a softer touch.*

difficulty
easy

minimum hair length
top of shoulders

what you'll need
hair clips

large-barrel (1½ in.; 35mm)
curling wand or iron

clear small elastic (or a color
that matches your hair)

hairspray

1 Separate out a section from your front hairline to your crown for the mohawk. Clip away, and then create beach waves.

Create as narrow or wide a section as desired

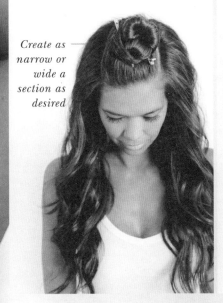

2 Create a French braid using the mohawk section. Finish the bottom of the French braid with a basic braid. Secure with an elastic.

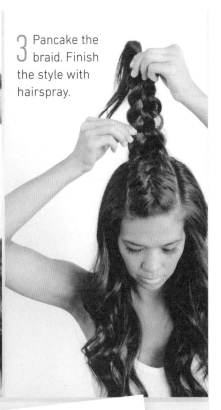

3 Pancake the braid. Finish the style with hairspray.

style tip

If you're wanting an even fuller, more dramatic look, you can lightly tease the entire mohawk section prior to creating the French braid, as well as the hair hanging down on the sides and the back after curling. Just be careful not to overtease the hair.

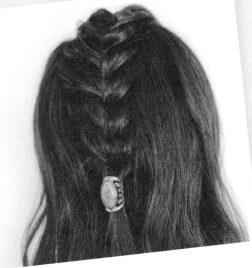

accessorize it!
Run the braid through any enormous, ornate rings you own, and then bobby pin the back of the ring vertically up toward the braid to keep it in place.

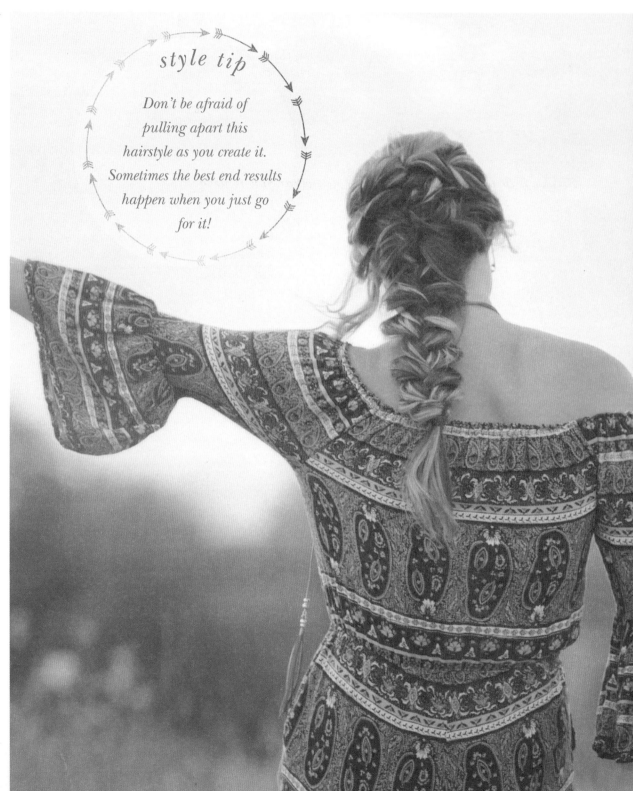

love
KNOT

*Believe it or not, this impressive style—with its appearance of **loose knots**—revolves around a simple **French braid.** Great for a day when you're in a hurry, you can throw it together and walk out the door looking effortlessly beautiful.*

difficulty
intermediate

minimum hair length
shoulder blades

what you'll need
large-barrel (1 ½ in.; 35mm) curling wand or iron
hair clips
clear small elastics (or a color that matches your hair)
bobby pins
hairspray

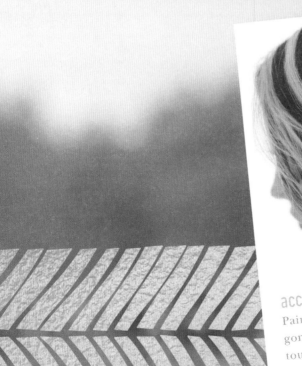

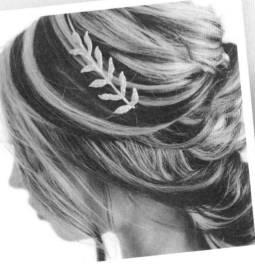

accessorize it!
Pair your favorite headband with this gorgeous hairstyle. This simple yet elegant touch will make the front of it even more appealing.

1 Create beach waves. Separate your hair into three sections, similar to a mohawk, and clip each section.

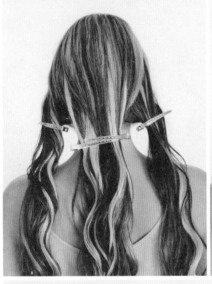

2 French braid the middle section. Secure the end with an elastic.

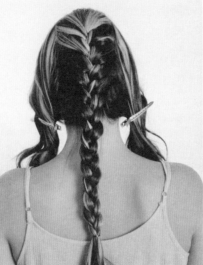

3 At the front of the right side, pull out a medium-size section. Twist the section up and over toward the back.

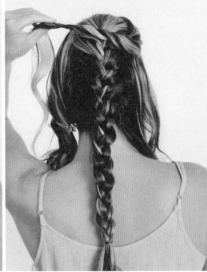

4 Wrap and tuck the twist into the first crossings of the French braid, leaving the tail sticking out.

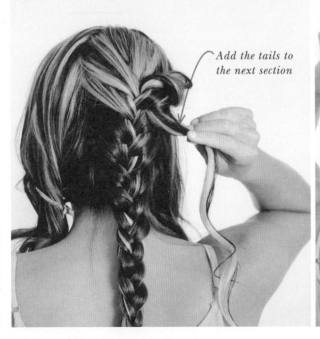

Add the tails to the next section

5 Repeat steps 3 and 4 using hair from the left side.

Add the tails to the next section

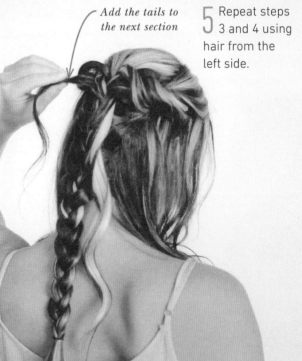

6 On each side, continue taking medium-size sections and twisting them up and toward the back. Wrap and tuck them into the middle of the braid.

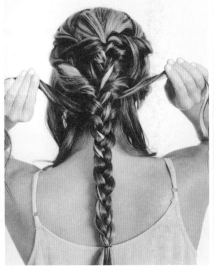

7 Once you reach the bottom half of the braid, tuck the longer tails from the previous sections into the lower parts of the braid. Secure the leftover tails to the bottom of the braid with an elastic.

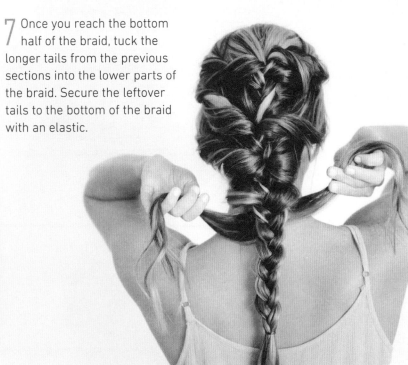

8 Loosen up the twists and secure any extra loose pieces with bobby pins. Finish the style with hairspray.

Slide the bobby pin through the twist

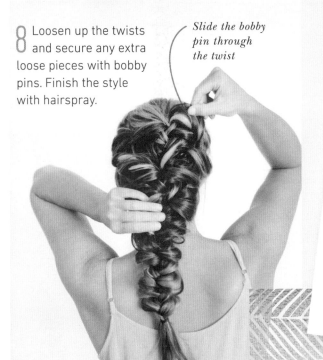

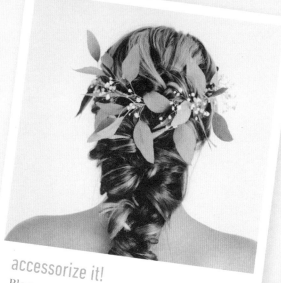

accessorize it!

Place a crown of delicate eucalyptus leaves and baby's breath around the top of the hairstyle.

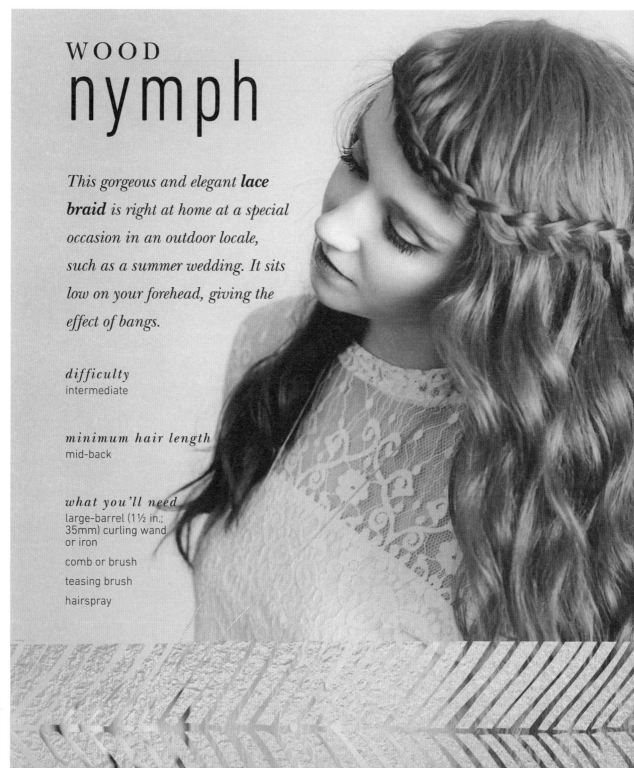

WOOD
nymph

This gorgeous and elegant **lace braid** is right at home at a special occasion in an outdoor locale, such as a summer wedding. It sits low on your forehead, giving the effect of bangs.

difficulty
intermediate

minimum hair length
mid-back

what you'll need
large-barrel (1 ½ in.; 35mm) curling wand or iron

comb or brush

teasing brush

hairspray

1 Create beach waves. Part your hair deep to one side.

2 Working on the heavy side of the part, start a Dutch braid, adding in hair only from the top.

3 Continue braiding across your forehead, pancaking the bottom edge as you go. Once you get to the end of the part, stop adding in hair.

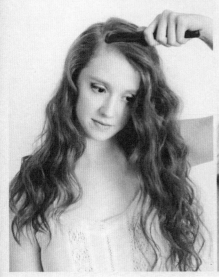

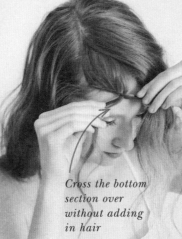

Cross the bottom section over without adding in hair

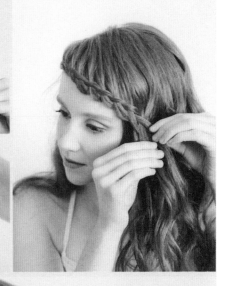

style tip

When braiding across your forehead, your hair will tend to want to spring up a little once finished due to its natural volume. To compensate for this, work on the braid a little lower than you want it to sit while placing the hand you hold the braid with right where you want the braid to sit.

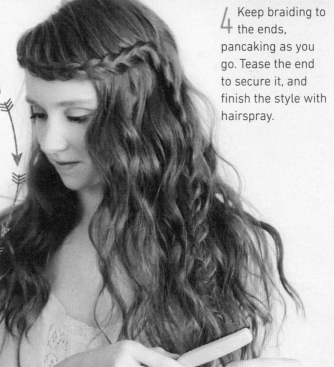

4 Keep braiding to the ends, pancaking as you go. Tease the end to secure it, and finish the style with hairspray.

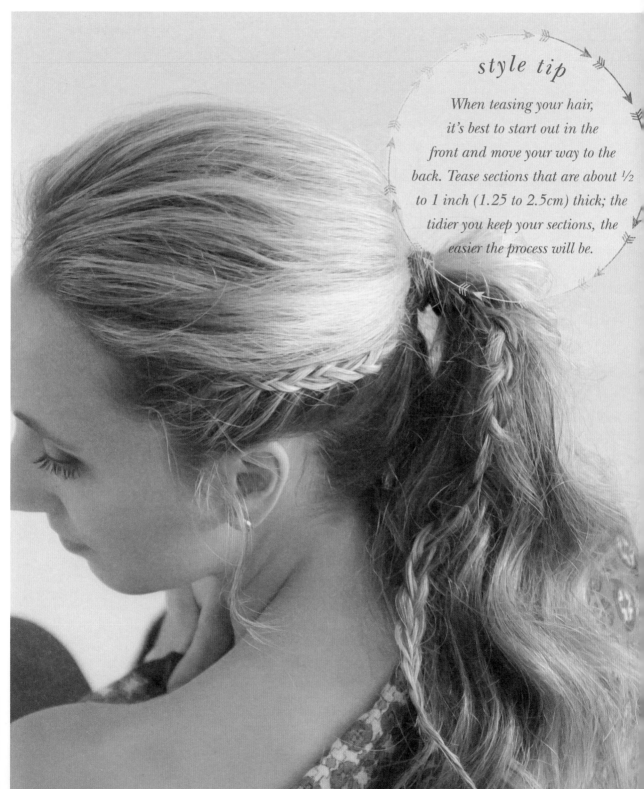

style tip

When teasing your hair, it's best to start out in the front and move your way to the back. Tease sections that are about ½ to 1 inch (1.25 to 2.5cm) thick; the tidier you keep your sections, the easier the process will be.

fierce
AND FUN

*Looking for a ponytail with attitude? This **edgy style** incorporates **a braid** to take your appearance up a notch. Whether you're planning to hit the gym or to go out with friends, you get a look with a certain je ne sais quoi.*

what you'll need
large-barrel (1 ½ in.; 35mm) curling wand or iron
comb
hair clip
clear small elastic (or a color that matches your hair)
teasing brush
clear ponytail elastic (or a color that matches your hair)
bobby pins
hairspray

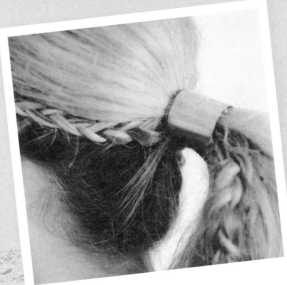

accessorize it!
Instead of wrapping the ponytail with a section of your hair, accessorize it with a ponytail cuff.

1 Create beach waves. Make a part from about 1½ inches (3.75cm) above your ear to the nape of your neck.

Clip the hair on top so it's out of the way

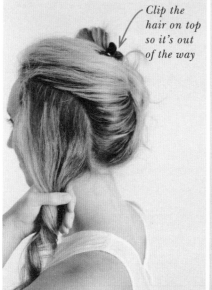

2 Split the hair below the part into three sections. Make a lace braid, adding in hair only from the section closest to your ear.

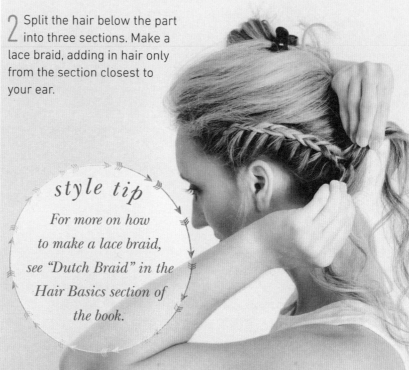

style tip

For more on how to make a lace braid, see "Dutch Braid" in the Hair Basics section of the book.

3 When you run out of hair to add, continue with a basic braid to the ends. Secure the bottom by teasing, or finish with an elastic.

Pancake the braid for more texture

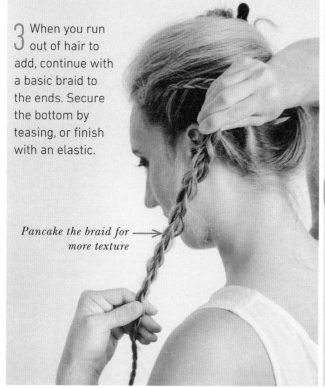

4 Tease the hair at the crown of your head, starting about 2 inches (5cm) from your hairline and finishing about 3 inches (7.5cm) back.

Smooth the front hair back gently with your brush

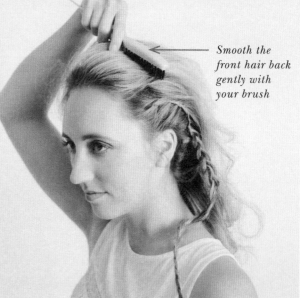

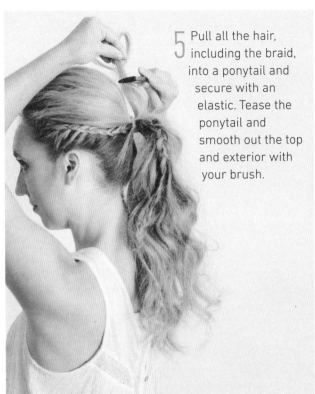

5 Pull all the hair, including the braid, into a ponytail and secure with an elastic. Tease the ponytail and smooth out the top and exterior with your brush.

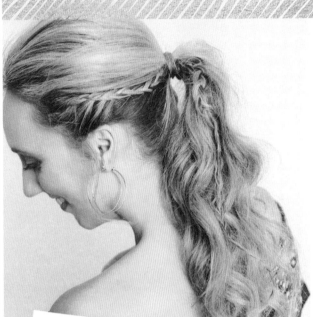

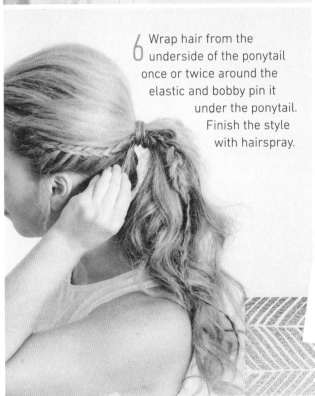

6 Wrap hair from the underside of the ponytail once or twice around the elastic and bobby pin it under the ponytail. Finish the style with hairspray.

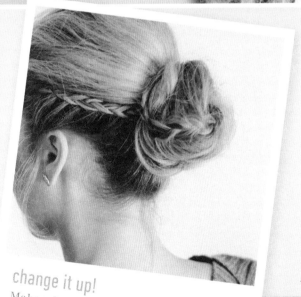

change it up!

Make a bun out of the ponytail, wrap the base of the bun with the braid, and pin in place.

fierce AND FUN 55

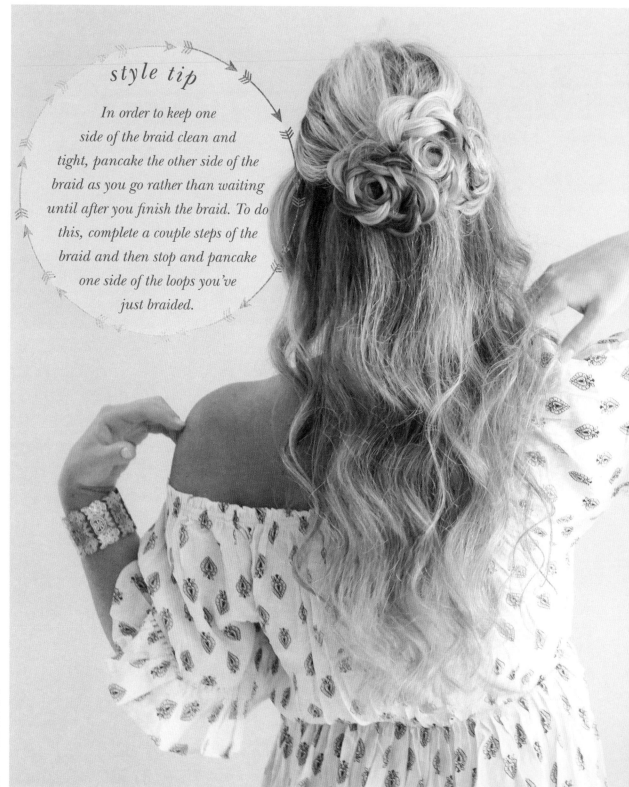

style tip

In order to keep one side of the braid clean and tight, pancake the other side of the braid as you go rather than waiting until after you finish the braid. To do this, complete a couple steps of the braid and then stop and pancake one side of the loops you've just braided.

flower
POWER

*This flowery style has a **delicate, elegant feel** that's just right for more formal occasions, such as a wedding or prom. Even though it appears complex, it's **surprisingly easy** to put together and looks great on most hair types and textures.*

difficulty
easy

minimum hair length
mid-back

what you'll need
clear small elastics (or a color that matches your hair)
teasing comb
bobby pins

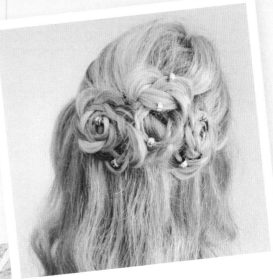

accessorize it!
Attach hair clips randomly in the "petals" of the flowers to add more romance to the style.

1 Divide the top of your hair into three ponytails at the back and secure with elastics. Make sure to leave hair loose over your ears.

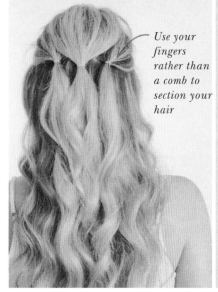

Use your fingers rather than a comb to section your hair

2 Using the middle ponytail, begin a basic braid. As you braid, pancake one side while leaving the other side tight. Tease the hair to secure it.

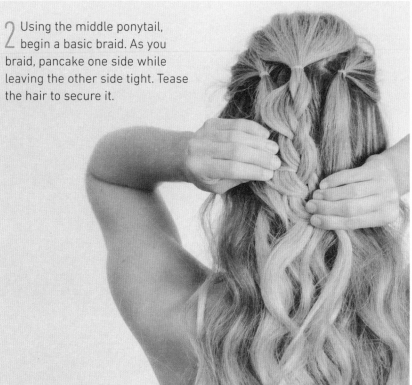

3 Starting at the bottom, roll the braid up toward the tight side of the braid to make a flower bun. Secure against your crown with bobby pins.

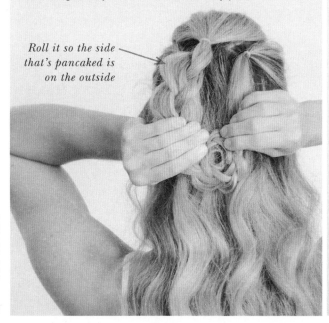

Roll it so the side that's pancaked is on the outside

4 With the remaining ponytails, repeat steps 2 and 3. Pin the new flowers next to the middle one.

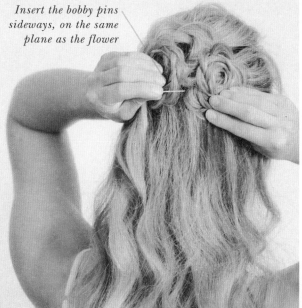

Insert the bobby pins sideways, on the same plane as the flower

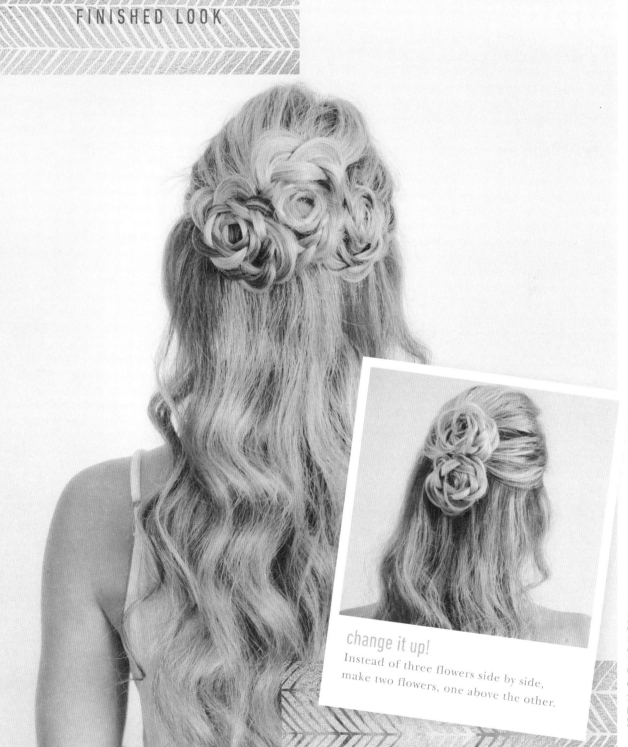

change it up!
Instead of three flowers side by side, make two flowers, one above the other.

secret
GARDEN

*This is truly a style for beginners, as it doesn't require any actual braiding. By using elastics and twists, you create a **lovely faux braid** that stays put without coming apart. Wear it on a girls' night out or at a casual get-together.*

difficulty
easy

minimum hair length
mid-back

what you'll need
brush
clear ponytail elastics (or a color that matches your hair)

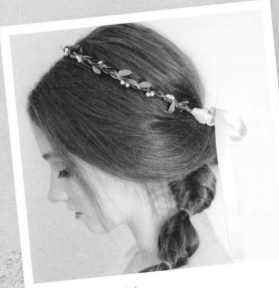

accessorize it!
Embrace your inner hippe by adding a flower crown.

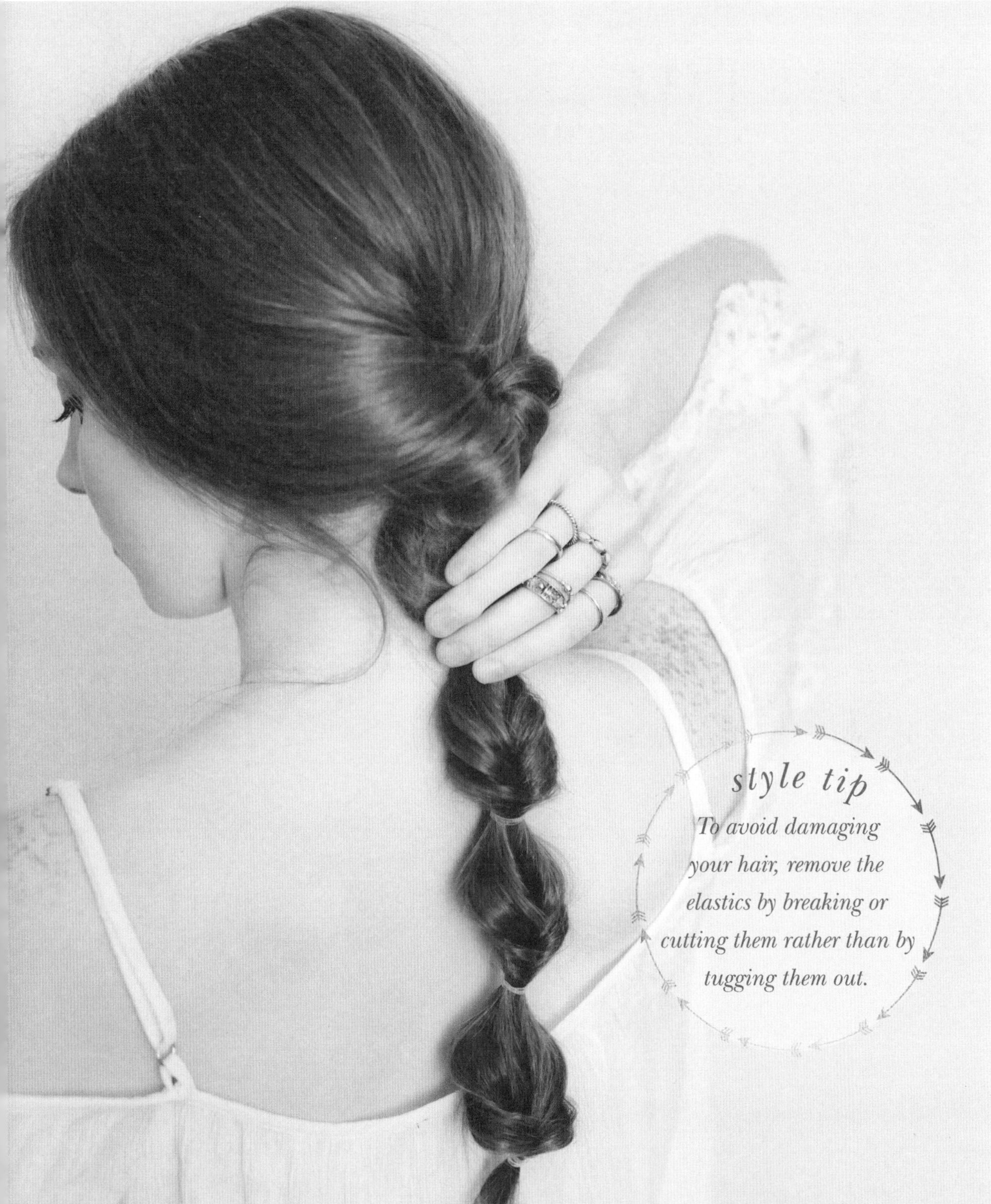

style tip

To avoid damaging your hair, remove the elastics by breaking or cutting them rather than by tugging them out.

1 Gather all of your hair into a loose, low ponytail at the back of your head and secure with an elastic.

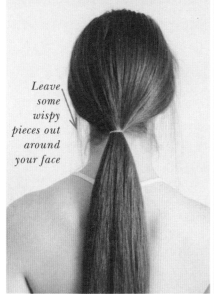

Leave some wispy pieces out around your face

2 Split the hair above the elastic in half by reaching up the middle with your thumb and index fingers.

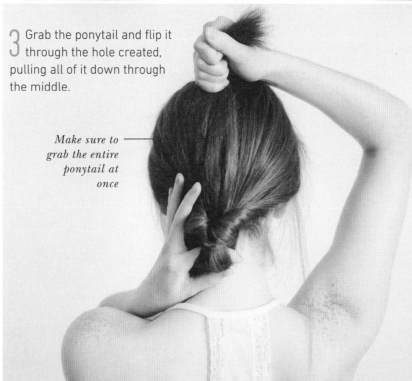

3 Grab the ponytail and flip it through the hole created, pulling all of it down through the middle.

Make sure to grab the entire ponytail at once

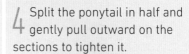

4 Split the ponytail in half and gently pull outward on the sections to tighten it.

Don't tug too hard; it can make the top messy

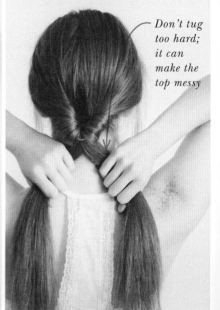

5 Gently pull the twisted hair above the elastic looser to fill in the gap above the elastic and to add volume.

6 Place an elastic about 2 to 3 inches (5 to 7.5cm) below the ponytail and reach through the middle again. Flip the ponytail through the hole.

7 Gently pull the twisted hair above the elastic looser to fill in the gap above the elastic and to add volume. Repeat steps 6 and 7 until you run out of hair.

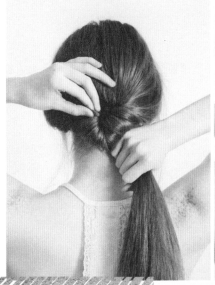

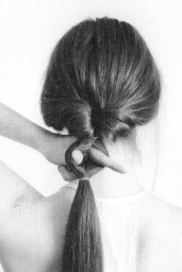

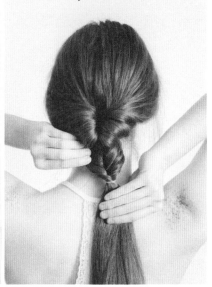

FINISHED
LOOK

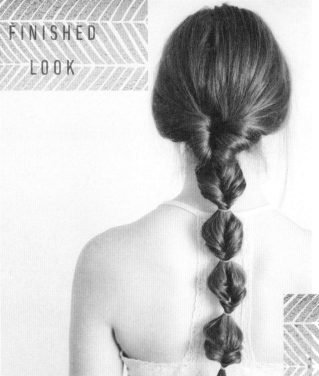

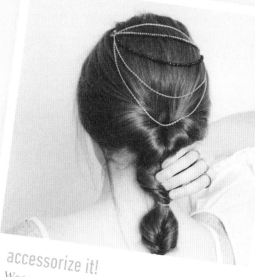

accessorize it!
Wear a clip-in hair chain centered above the braid to enhance its dreamy appearance.

7 STYLES FOR THE DARING

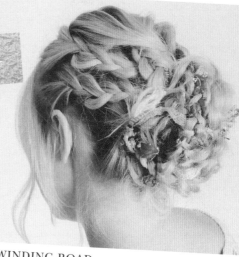

WINDING ROAD
Although this style is simply made up of basic braids, only a bold gal would weave in all of the ribbons.

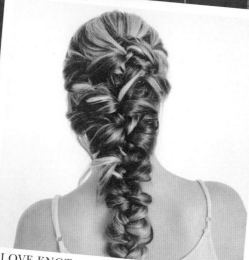

LOVE KNOT
This style is perfect for the girl who's willing to take her French braid to the next level.

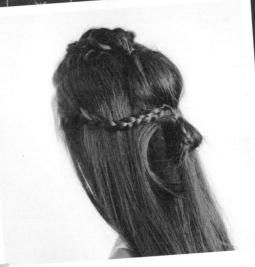

WILD CHILD
A mohawk, a half-bun, and side braids—this style brings together everything you could want.

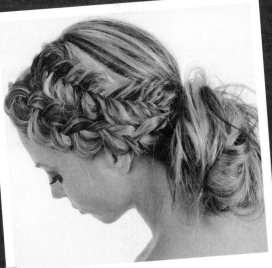

ORNATE RINGS
The more braids, the more spunkiness you show off. Wearing two types of braids in one hairstyle says it all!

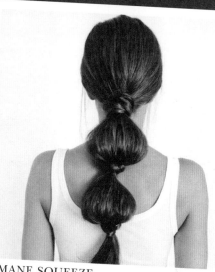

MANE SQUEEZE
If you're looking to make a statement, this bubble ponytail gives the traditional style a funky twist.

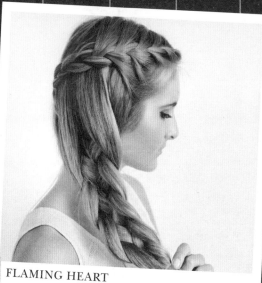

FLAMING HEART
Only a true braid lover would be brazen enough to try this gorgeous five-strand braid.

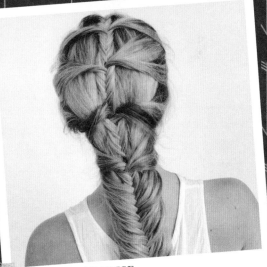

HIDDEN PARADISE
Are you ready for layers and fishtails? This isn't your mama's braid. You've gotta have guts to wear this style!

gentle
WATERFALL

If a hairstyle can be soothing, this braid captures such **calmness**. *The waterfall braid is well known for its complexity, so it requires great attention to detail on your part. However, the* **unique** *and* **versatile** *final result is sure to impress.*

difficulty
challenging

minimum hair length
top of shoulders

what you'll need
large-barrel (1½ in.; 35mm) curling wand or iron
clear small elastics (or a color that matches your hair)
hairspray

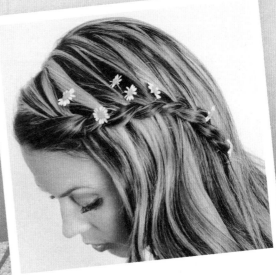

accessorize it!
Finish this style off with a few flowers pinned along the braid to give it an extra-romantic touch.

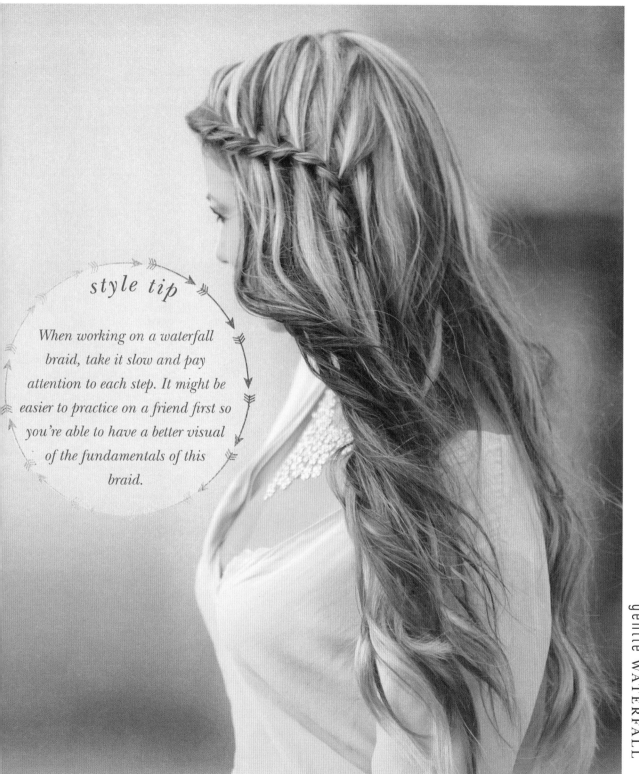

style tip

When working on a waterfall braid, take it slow and pay attention to each step. It might be easier to practice on a friend first so you're able to have a better visual of the fundamentals of this braid.

1 Create beach waves. Divide the first layer of hair on one side of your head into three small sections.

The sectioning is similar to the start of a French braid

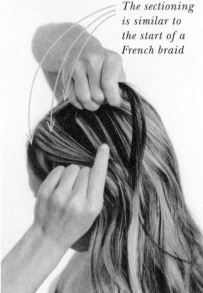

2 Cross the right section over the middle section.

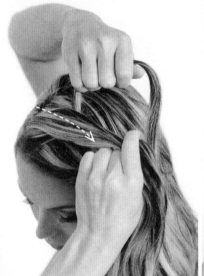

3 Cross the left section over the middle section you created in step 2.

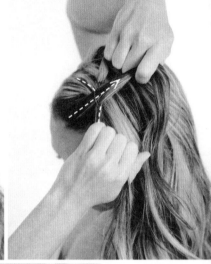

4 Cross the right section over the middle section.

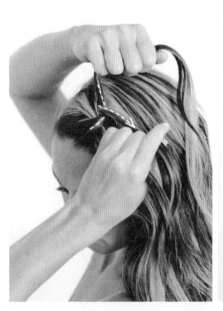

5 Take a new section from the top near your part, follow the section you crossed over in step 4, and release it.

This section remains out of the braid

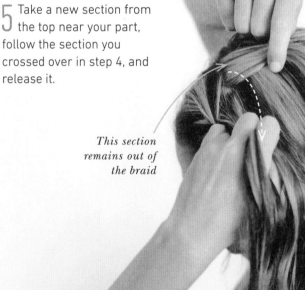

6 Cross the left section over the middle section. Next, cross the right section over the middle section.

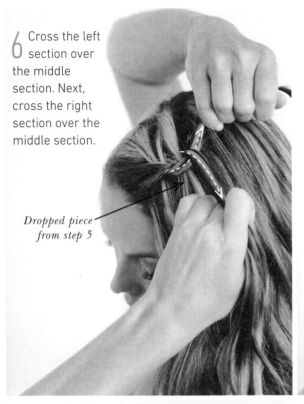

Dropped piece from step 5

7 Take a new section from the top near your part, follow the section you crossed over in step 6, and release it.

This section remains out of the braid

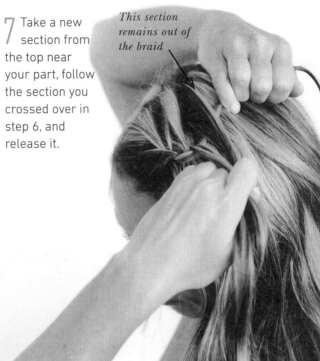

8 Repeat the crossover and release process until you reach the back. Finish off with a basic braid and then secure with an elastic. Finish the style with hairspray.

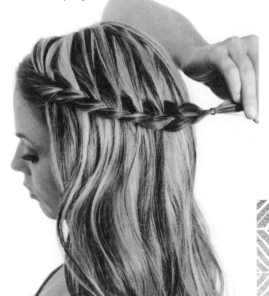

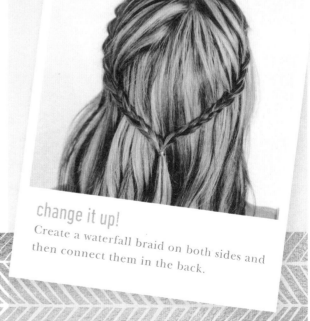

change it up!

Create a waterfall braid on both sides and then connect them in the back.

WHIMSICAL
roots

*A **tangle of braids** is paired with a **loose, swept-back, half-up** style to create this laid-back look. The nice thing is, you can make it as messy as you want. Feel free to experiment with the placement of your braid "roots" and see what you think looks best.*

difficulty
easy

minimum hair length
top of shoulders

what you'll need
clear small elastics (or a color that matches your hair)
bobby pins
hairspray

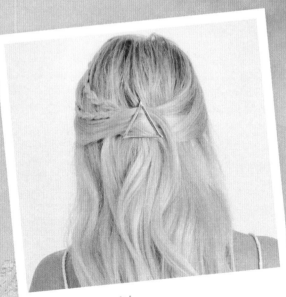

accessorize it!
After completing the hairstyle, attach a triangle clip, where all the bobby pins are, to really unify the style.

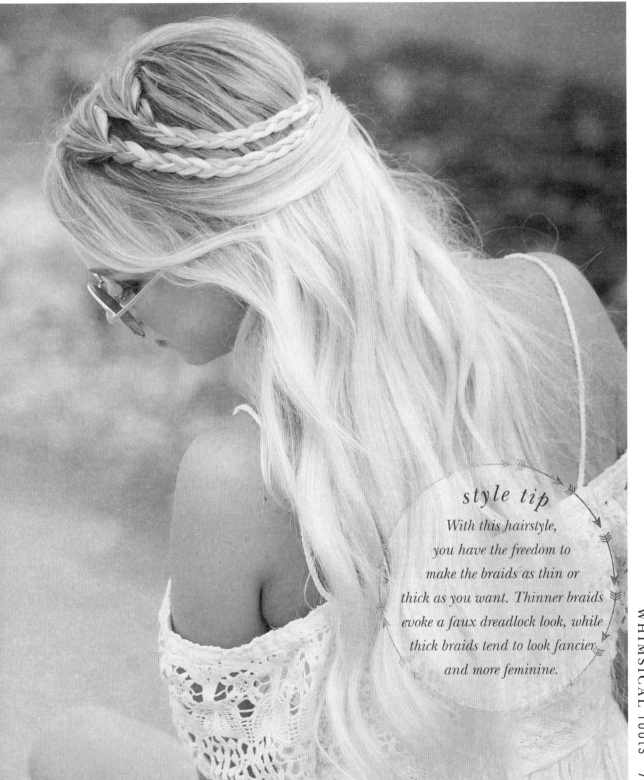

style tip

With this hairstyle,
you have the freedom to
make the braids as thin or
thick as you want. Thinner braids
evoke a faux dreadlock look, while
thick braids tend to look fancier
and more feminine.

1 Starting with a side part, create two slender basic braids on the heavier side of the part. Secure each with an elastic.

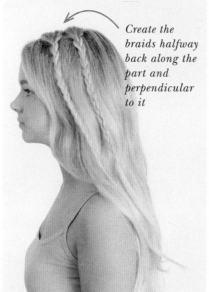

Create the braids halfway back along the part and perpendicular to it

2 Pin the braids together at the center of the back of your head, sliding the bobby pins directly into the braid sideways.

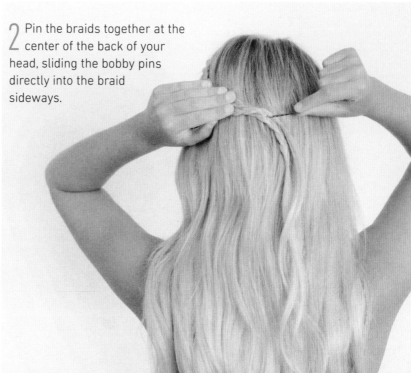

3 Take a section of hair from each side of your head, leaving out the hair immediately around your face.

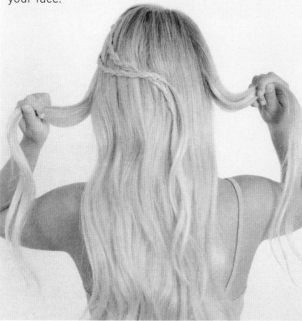

4 Drape the side sections below the braids and cross them over each other in the back.

Cover the bobby pins holding the braids

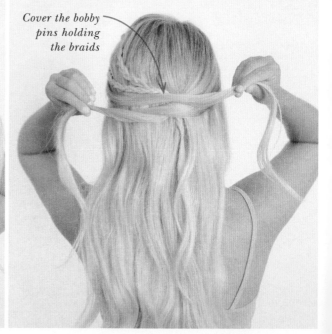

5 Secure the side sections right over the braids by sliding bobby pins sideways into your hair.

Slide bobby pins across and underneath the sections

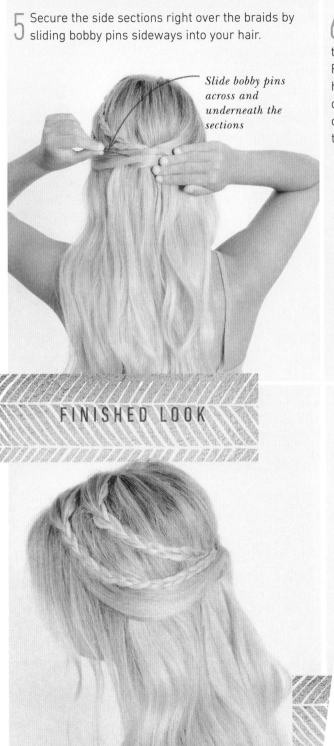

6 Cut out the elastics and unravel the tails of both braids. Finish the style with hairspray sprayed directly onto the crossed pieces in the back.

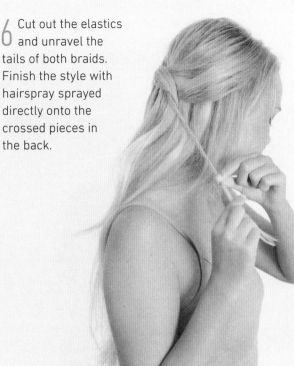

FINISHED LOOK

change it up!

Braid all the hair in the back into two loose basic braids that go halfway down the length of your hair. Connect them with a single elastic, and then wrap the elastic with a small strand of hair.

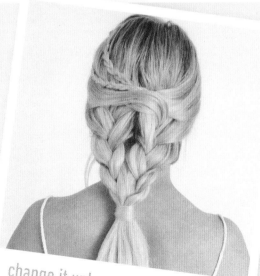

sun
GODDESS

Shine like a goddess with this romantic style, in which **crisscrossing braids** *sit atop a* **messy bun.** *Wear it to any summery event—from a formal event to an afternoon party—and bask in the admiration of those around you.*

difficulty
easy

minimum hair length
shoulder blades

what you'll need
hair clips
clear small elastics (or a color that matches your hair)
clear ponytail elastic (or a color that matches your hair)
bobby pins
hairspray

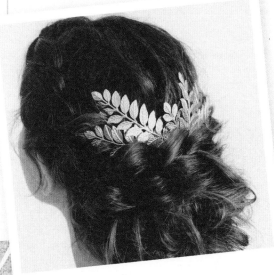

accessorize it!
Slide a leafy comb behind the braids so the leaves are visible, yet still tucked into the updo, for a delicate touch.

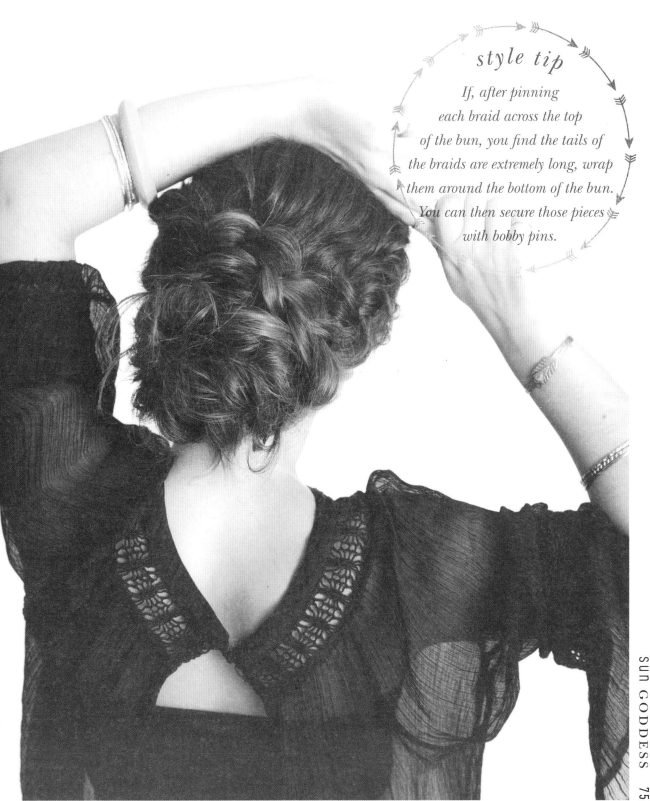

style tip

*If, after pinning
each braid across the top
of the bun, you find the tails of
the braids are extremely long, wrap
them around the bottom of the bun.
You can then secure those pieces
with bobby pins.*

SUN GODDESS 75

1 Use your fingers to part your hair to one side. Separate the hair on the back of your head from the hair on each side of the part.

Clip the three sections to keep them separate

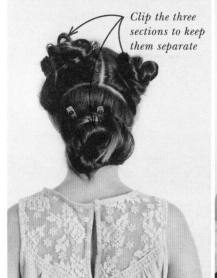

2 Create a Dutch braid on each side section, leaving out the hair on the crown so you have a soft-looking part. Secure each with an elastic.

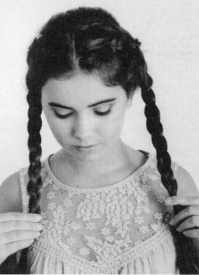

3 Place the hair from both the back and the crown into a ponytail. Secure with an elastic.

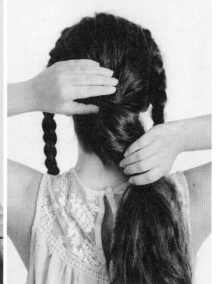

4 Loosely twist and wrap the ponytail to create a messy bun. Secure with bobby pins.

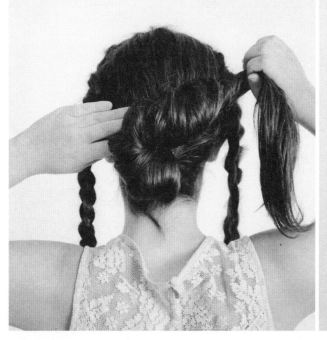

5 Pancake both Dutch braids to make them appear fuller.

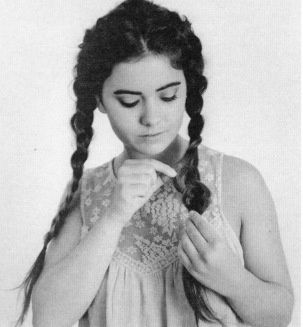

6 Drape the thinner of the Dutch braids across the top of the bun. Secure with bobby pins, sliding them sideways toward the hair.

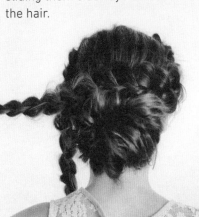

7 Drape the thicker braid on top of the smaller braid and wrap it around the bottom to hide the ends. Secure with bobby pins.

Hide the elastics under the braids

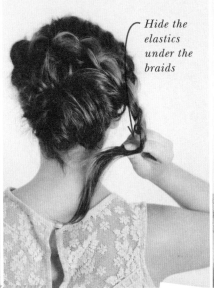

8 Loosen the crown area by gently pulling the hair up. Finish the style with hairspray.

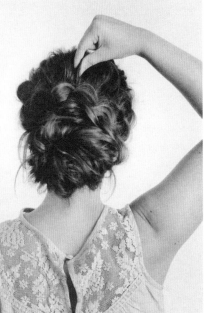

FINISHED LOOK

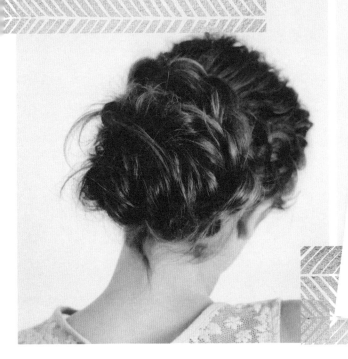

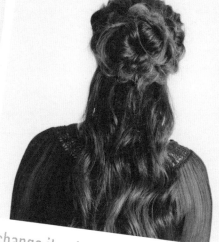

change it up!

Create a half-up style by leaving out the unbraided back section of hair and only using the hair from the crown of your head to create the ponytail.

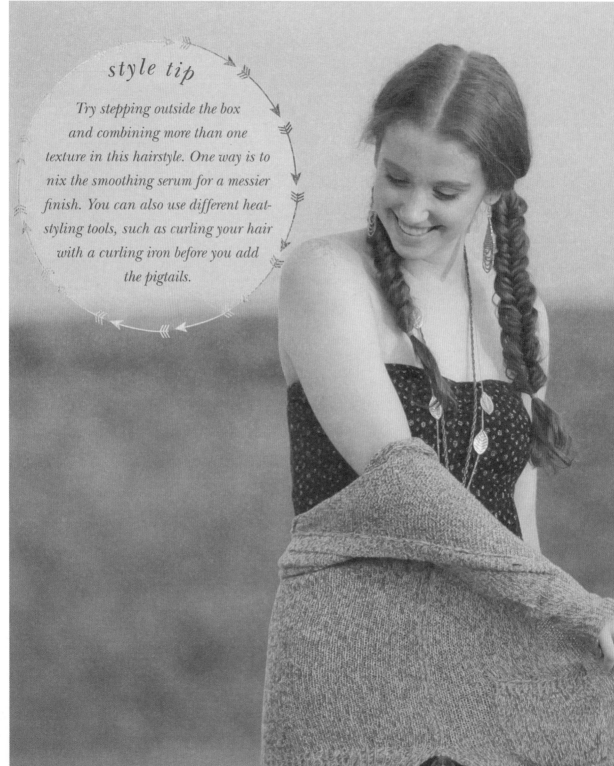

style tip

Try stepping outside the box and combining more than one texture in this hairstyle. One way is to nix the smoothing serum for a messier finish. You can also use different heat-styling tools, such as curling your hair with a curling iron before you add the pigtails.

hippie
CARAVAN

This hairstyle, which combines a **sleek crown** *with* **textured pigtails,** *is a throwback to the summer of love. It's great for beating the heat at concerts and other summertime events. While best done on clean, dry, and straight hair, these pigtails can work on other hair textures as well.*

difficulty
easy

minimum hair length
mid-back

what you'll need
comb
flatiron
smoothing serum
clear small elastics (or a color that matches your hair)
dry shampoo

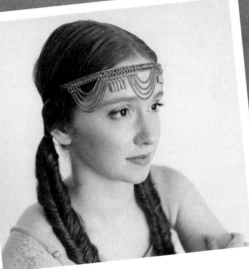

accessorize it!
Add a hippie headband to really capture that feeling of summer.

1 Flatiron your hair, focusing on the roots.

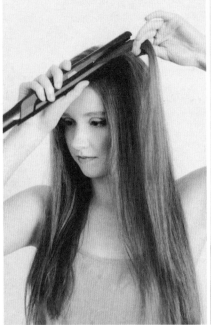

2 Use a comb to part your hair down the middle, from the front all the way down to the nape of your neck.

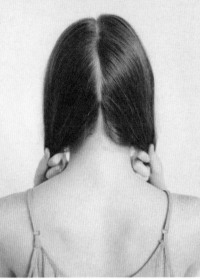

3 Put your hair into low pigtails directly behind your ears and secure with elastics. Make sure to leave the tops of your ears covered.

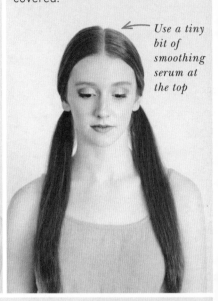

Use a tiny bit of smoothing serum at the top

4 To create texture and fullness, spray each pigtail with dry shampoo and finger comb it through your hair.

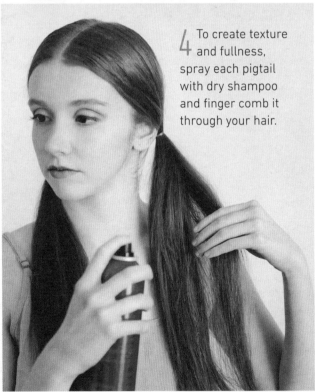

5 Fishtail braid each pigtail, going as close to the ends of your hair as possible. Secure each with an elastic.

Bring in small sections

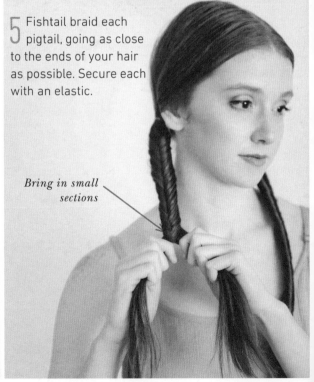

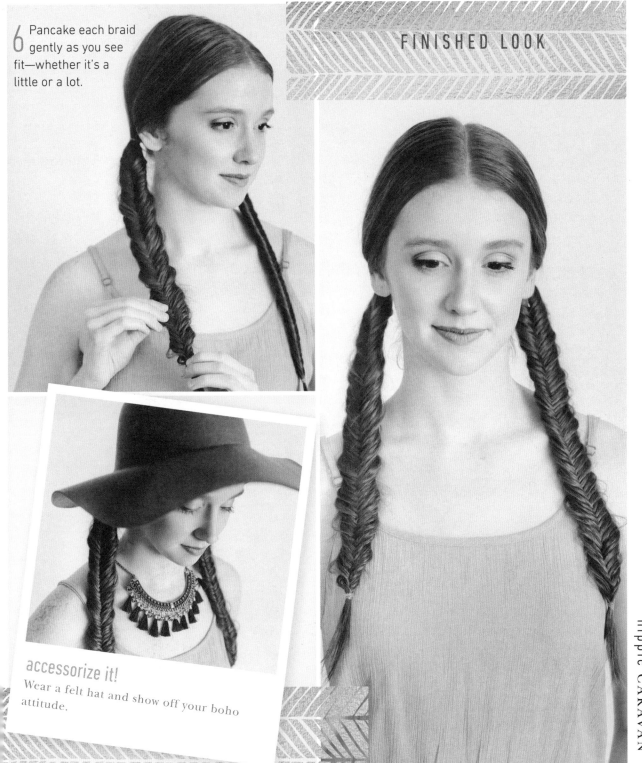

6 Pancake each braid gently as you see fit—whether it's a little or a lot.

accessorize it!

Wear a felt hat and show off your boho attitude.

MERMAID
tail

If you want to feel like a mermaid—no swimming required—this hairstyle is sure to do just that! The **long, relaxed waves** *and* **herringbone braid** *combine to create a cute, casual look that'd fit right in at the pool or on the beach.*

difficulty
intermediate

minimum hair length
top of shoulders

what you'll need
large-barrel (1 ½ in.; 35mm) curling wand or iron
hair clips
three-clip clip-in hair extension weft
clear small elastic (or a color that matches your hair)
bobby pins
hairspray

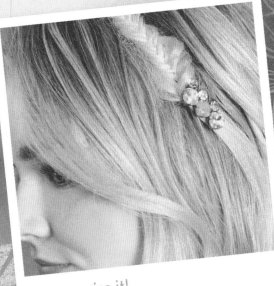

accessorize it!
Hold the band in place with three small pins. It's fun and also provides extra security for the braid.

To help the braid
stay in place, right before
you wrap the braid across, spray
a firm-hold hairspray on the
underside of the braid, as well as the
area where the braid will lie on
top of your head.

1 Create beach waves. Separate and clip away the entire crown area of hair on your head.

2 Apply the three-clip hair extension weft to the section of hair underneath the sectioned-off crown area.

3 Gently pull the hair extension and a small amount of your natural hair together toward the right side.

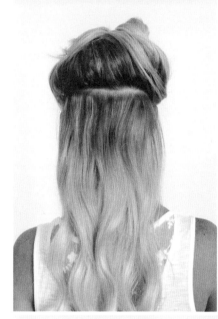
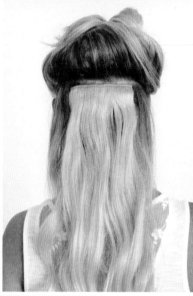
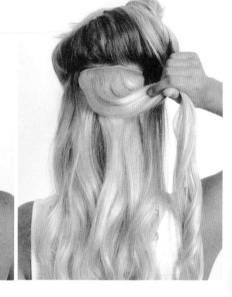

4 Use that hair to create a fishtail braid. Secure the end with an elastic, and then pancake the braid.

5 Wrap the fishtail across the top of your head. Secure the end of it by crisscrossing the bobby pins behind your ear.

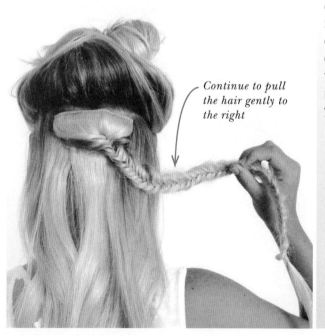

Continue to pull the hair gently to the right

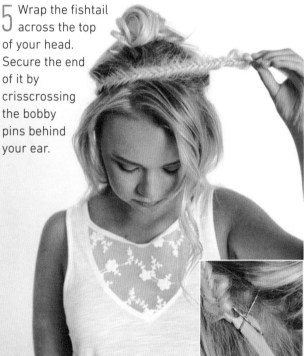

6 Remove the hair clip from the crown area, letting the hair fall to cover the bobby pins and extensions track. Place bobby pins throughout the braid so it doesn't slide backward. Finish the style with hairspray.

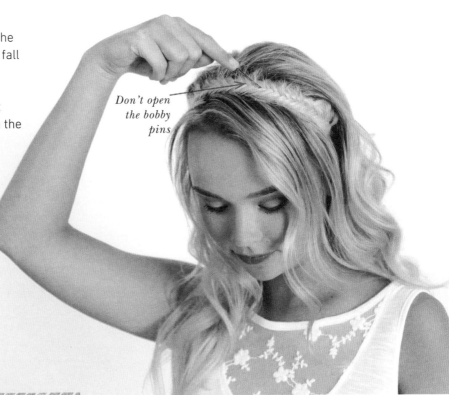

Don't open the bobby pins

FINISHED LOOK

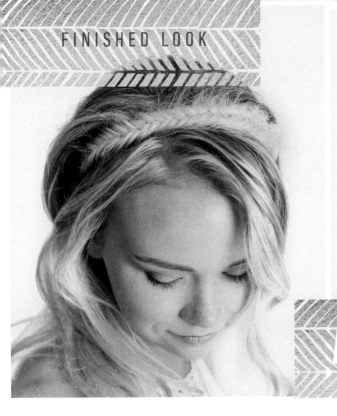

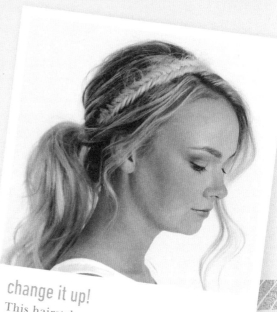

change it up!
This hairstyle transitions perfectly into a loose, low ponytail.

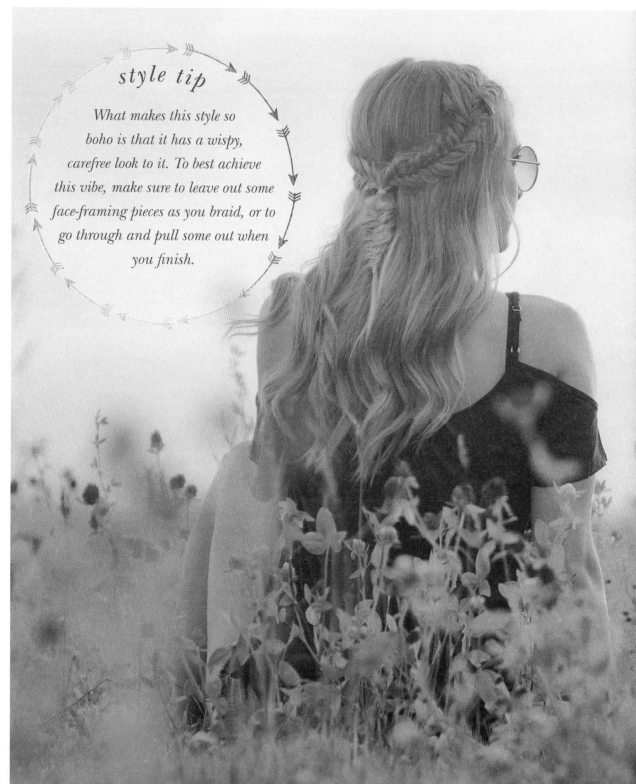

style tip

What makes this style so boho is that it has a wispy, carefree look to it. To best achieve this vibe, make sure to leave out some face-framing pieces as you braid, or to go through and pull some out when you finish.

FIELD OF
dreams

*Channel the feeling of a relaxed afternoon with this **half-up style.** Highly versatile, it can be worn as an informal 'do while you're playing tourist on vacation or dressed up with curls for a more formal event.*

difficulty
intermediate

minimum hair length
mid-back

what you'll need
brush
large-barrel (1 ½ in.; 35mm) curling wand or iron
clear small elastics (or a color that matches your hair)

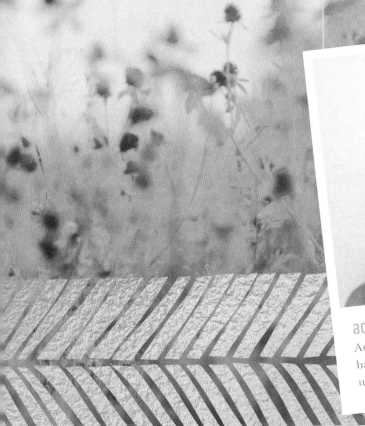

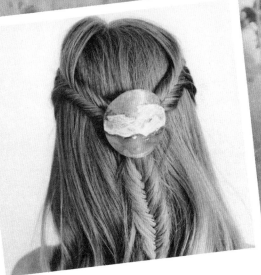

accessorize it!
Add a big barrette to hide the top elastic band, as well as to give the style a more unified appearance.

1 Create beach waves. Part your hair down the middle.

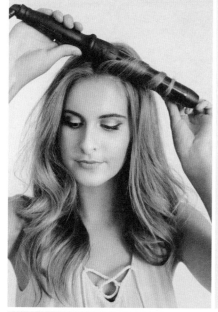

2 Starting with a triangular section at the front of your part, make a French fishtail on one side of your head, pancaking as you go.

Leave out some face-framing pieces as you braid →

3 When you get to your ear, stop adding in hair and fishtail braid to the ends. Secure with an elastic.

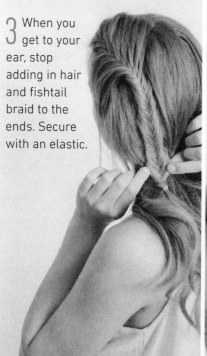

4 Repeat steps 2 and 3 on the opposite side of your head.

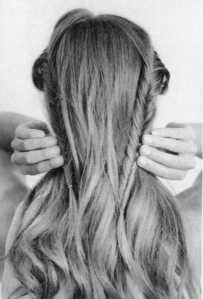

5 Join the two braids at the center of the back of your head with an elastic.

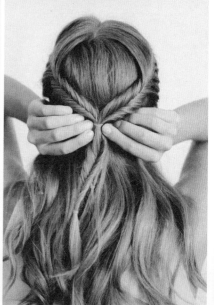

6 Break or cut the elastics securing the bottom of the two braids. Unbraid the two braids below the remaining elastic.

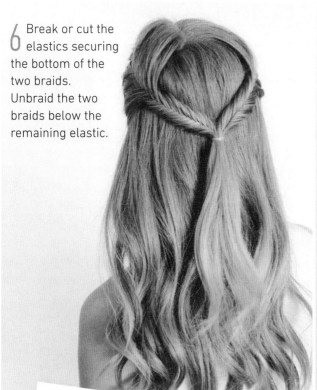

7 Join the two sections and fishtail braid all the way to the ends, pancaking as you go. Secure with an elastic.

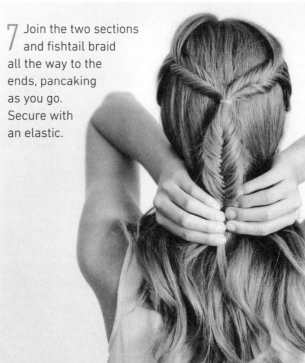

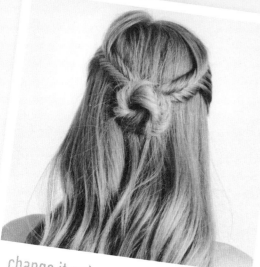

change it up!
Wrap the single fishtail braid into a bun that covers the top elastic band.

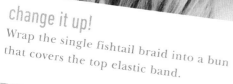

FINISHED LOOK

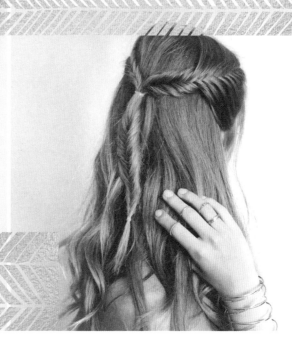

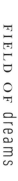

queen
OF HEARTS

Feel like royalty by wearing this **milkmaid-style braid.** *Despite its regal appearance, it's very easy to do, making it ideal for anytime you're in a rush to get out the door. This style truly allows you to embrace fashion and function.*

difficulty
easy

minimum hair length
mid-back

what you'll need
hair clips
clear small elastics (or a color that matches your hair)
bobby pins
hairspray

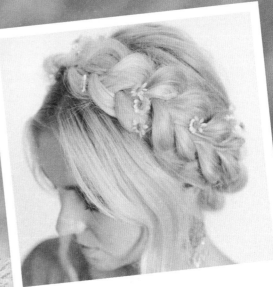

accessorize it!
For a touch of whimsy, add in small flowers throughout the braids. You can even mix different types of flowers or add greenery.

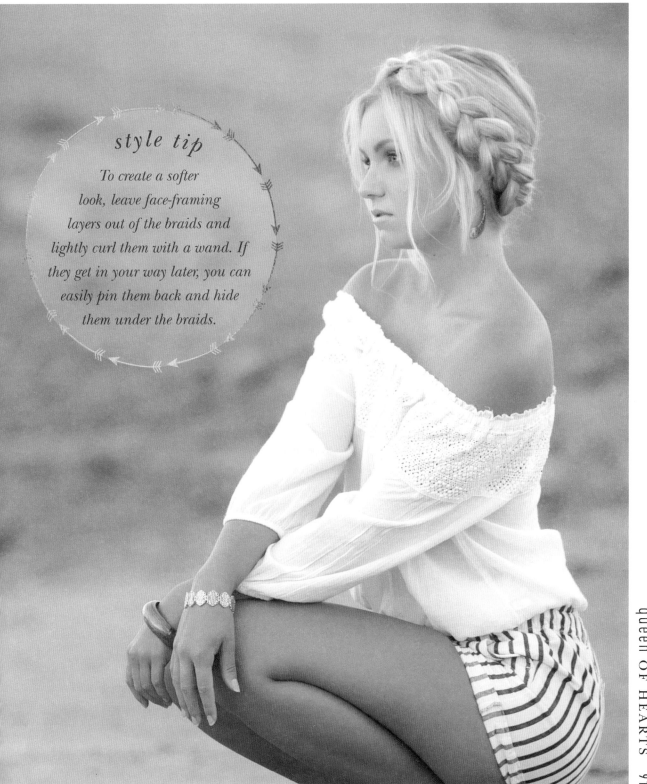

style tip

To create a softer
look, leave face-framing
layers out of the braids and
lightly curl them with a wand. If
they get in your way later, you can
easily pin them back and hide
them under the braids.

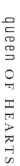

1 Separate your hair into two sections at the back hairline; don't make a straight part down the middle.

Use an equal amount of hair for each section

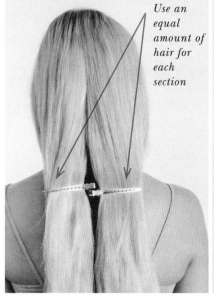

2 Put each section into a low basic braid, placing them as close as possible to the center. Secure each with an elastic.

3 Pancake each braid to make them fuller.

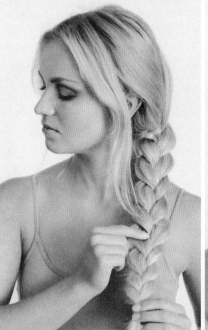

4 Bring the left braid under the right braid and wrap it around the right side of your head.

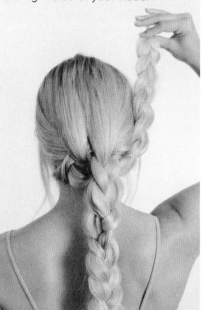

5 Secure the end of the left braid to the top of your head with crisscrossing bobby pins.

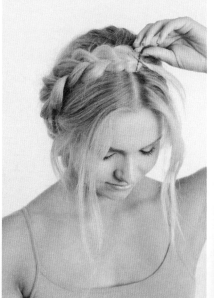

6 Bring the right braid to the left and wrap it around the left side of your head. Tuck the tail under the other braid and secure with bobby pins.

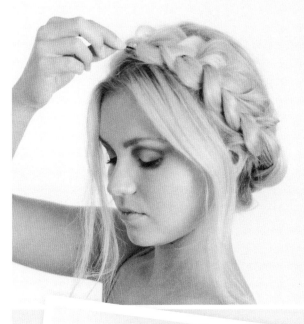

7 Loosen the loops of each braid. Slide bobby pins throughout the braids so the braids won't slip out of place. Finish the style with hairspray.

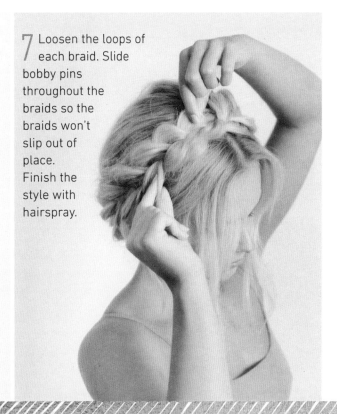

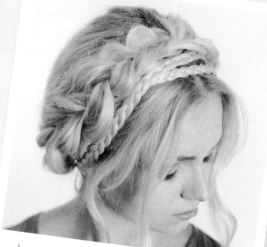

change it up!

Create two small basic braids, and then wrap and pin them next to the large braids for extra dimension.

FINISHED LOOK

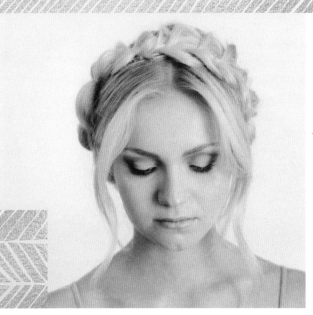

1 Divide your hair into two sections with a part that goes from the front hairline to the back hairline. Clip each section.

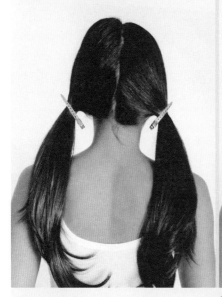

2 Unclip and create a Dutch braid on one side. Secure the end with an elastic. Repeat the process on the other side.

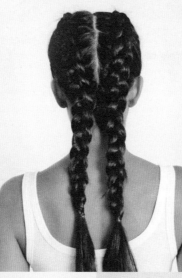

3 Beginning at the bottom and working your way upward, pancake the braids so they look chunkier.

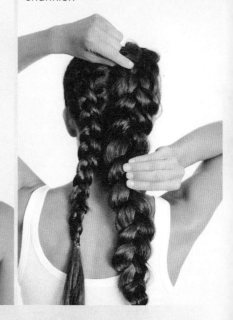

4 Bobby pin any loose loops. Finish the style with hairspray.

Slide bobby pins directly into the loop

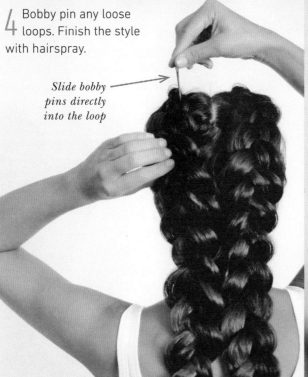

style tip

If your hair is layered, you may have a piece or two sticking out when you're finished pancaking the braids. No need to worry—boho is all about beautiful imperfection!

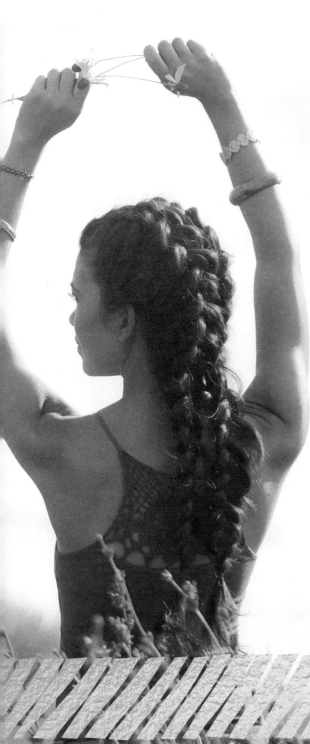

rapunzel

For this style, you really get to let down your hair. These **chunky Dutch braids** *will have everyone in awe of how thick your hair looks. To enhance the lushness, pancake as much as possible—the bigger the braids, the better!*

difficulty
intermediate

minimum hair length
waist

what you'll need
hair clips
clear small elastics (or a color that matches your hair)
hairspray

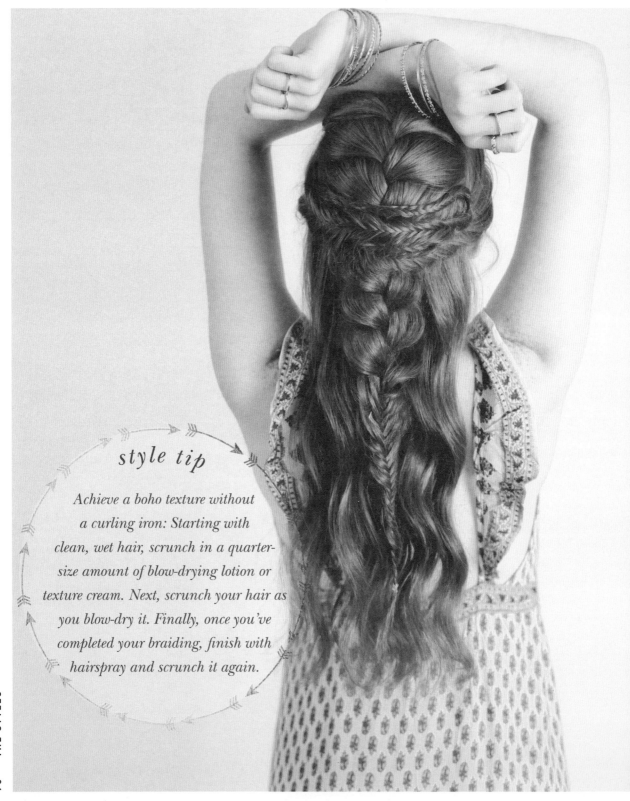

style tip

Achieve a boho texture without a curling iron: Starting with clean, wet hair, scrunch in a quarter-size amount of blow-drying lotion or texture cream. Next, scrunch your hair as you blow-dry it. Finally, once you've completed your braiding, finish with hairspray and scrunch it again.

MYSTICAL
maze

*This stunning, elaborate style will make you look like an expert braider. However, you only need to know **basic fishtail** and **French braids** to achieve it. Whether you dress it up or dress it down, you'll have a truly impressive style.*

difficulty
intermediate

minimum hair length
mid-back

what you'll need
large-barrel (1½ in.; 35mm) curling wand or iron

dry shampoo (optional)

bobby pins

clear small elastics (or a color that matches your hair)

teasing brush

hairspray

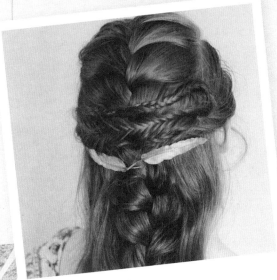

accessorize it!
Accentuate the fishtail braids by attaching a pair of brass feather barrettes right below them.

1 Create beach waves. If your hair is fine or silky, use dry shampoo to add texture.

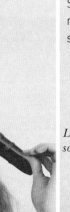

2 Finger comb your hair from the front to the back. Section out two pieces of hair right above your ears on each side. Pin them out of the way.

Leave out some face-framing pieces

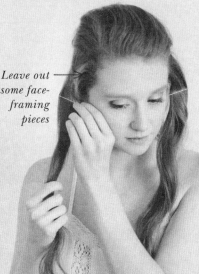

3 Starting at the front, French braid using large sections until you have half of your hair in the braid.

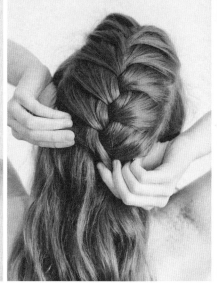

4 Switch to making a basic braid for 2 inches (5cm) and then secure with an elastic. Pancake the hair as much as possible.

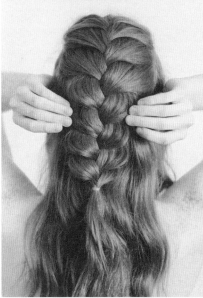

5 Using the loose hair below the elastic, make a fishtail braid. Secure with an elastic. Cut out the elastic between the two braids. Pancake the fishtail.

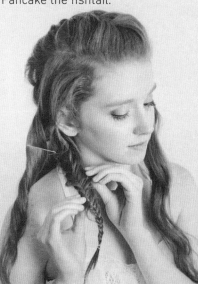

6 Make fishtail braids on each side of your head using the sections of hair from step 2. Tease the ends to secure them.

Pancake the braids as you make them

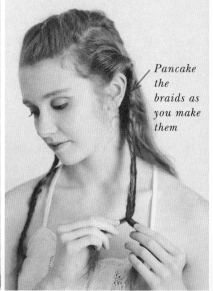

7 Take the fishtail braid on the right side across to the other side and pin it behind your ear.

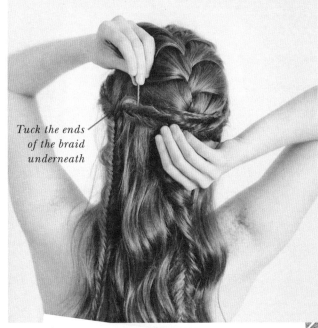

Tuck the ends of the braid underneath

8 Take the fishtail on the left side braid across to the right and pin it behind your ear. Finish the style with hairspray.

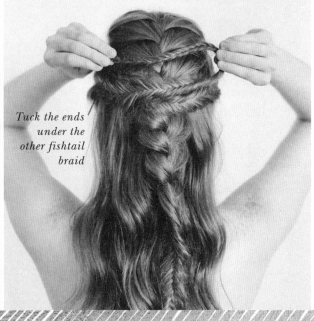

Tuck the ends under the other fishtail braid

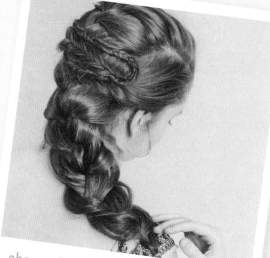

change it up!
Braid all of your loose hair into the French braid instead of only part of it.

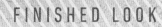

FINISHED LOOK

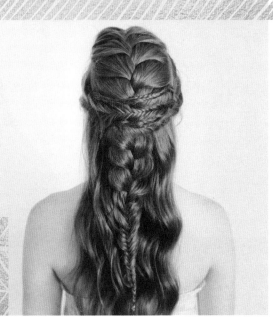

ORNATE
rings

*Mixing braids is always a fun way to spice up your hairstyle. In this look, a **Dutch braid** and an **ultra-textured fishtail braid** create "rings" around your head. Both braids are then combined into a **low, messy bun** for an extremely detailed boho style.*

difficulty
challenging

minimum hair length
shoulder blades

what you'll need
hair clips
clear small elastics (or a color that matches your hair)
clear ponytail elastics (or a color that matches your hair)
hairspray

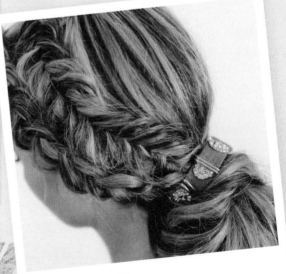

accessorize it!
Tie an embellished leather snap-on cuff—like what you would wear on your wrist—around the ponytail elastic to create a romantic bohemian look.

style tip

Loose strands are a good thing for this style. The trick for this bun is to leave the loose pieces as they fall and fight the urge to pin them away. Have fun with your hair and let it be free!

1 Create a deep side part. On the heavy side of the part, separate a section along your front hairline and clip it.

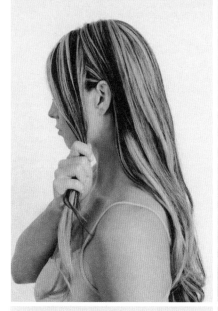

2 Section and clip a smaller section next to the first one.

This section is half the size of the front section

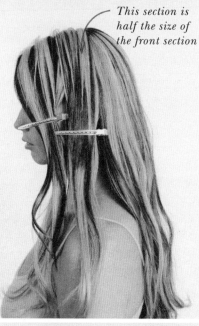

3 Create a Dutch braid using the section nearest your face. Secure with an elastic.

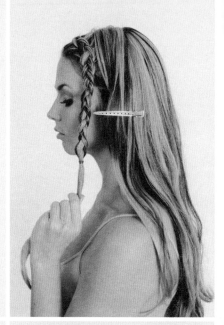

4 Create a fishtail braid using the smaller section. Secure with an elastic.

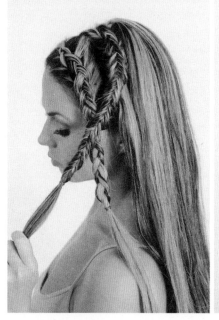

5 Pancake both braids to make them appear fuller.

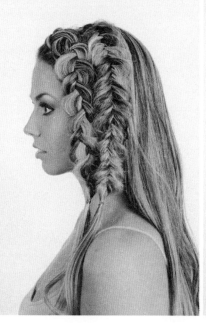

6 Place all of your hair, including the braids, into a low ponytail. Remove the elastics from both braids and undo the braids below the ponytail holder.

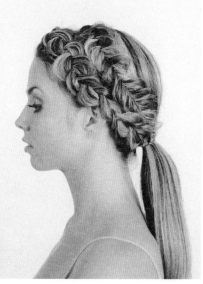

7 Place a second elastic around the existing ponytail and pull the ponytail only partway through.

8 Twist the elastic around the hair pulled through again while catching random strands in it to create the bun.

9 While holding the bun with one hand, loosen the crown area by gently pulling small areas up with your other hand. Finish the style with hairspray.

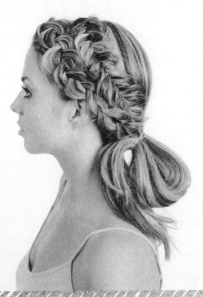

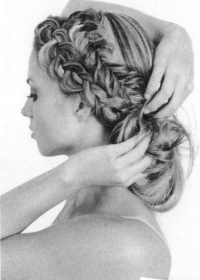

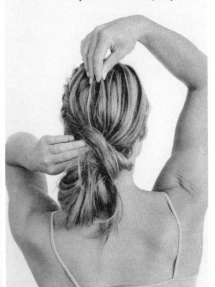

FINISHED LOOK

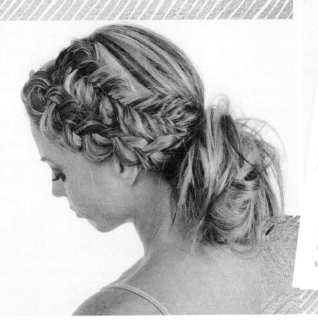

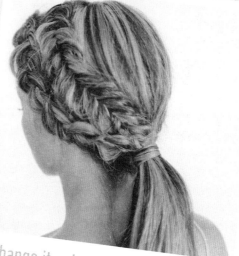

change it up!

Instead of placing your hair into a bun, leave it down in a ponytail, making sure to hide the elastic with a strand of hair wrapped around it.

7 STYLES YOU CAN DO IN 10 MINUTES

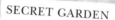

SECRET GARDEN
Don't have time for a real braid? This style uses a simple pull-through technique, so you'll be done in a snap.

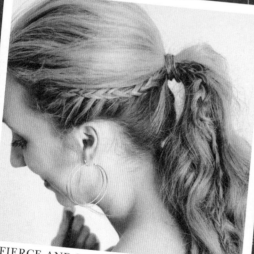

FIERCE AND FUN
If you're proficient at braiding, you can complete this simple braid and ponytail style very quickly.

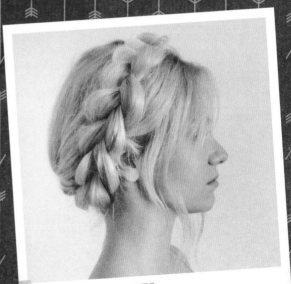

QUEEN OF HEARTS
Milkmaid braids, which consist of two basic braids, are super easy to do. You won't even need 10 minutes!

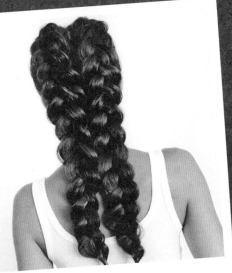

RAPUNZEL
Once you've mastered the Dutch braid, this will be your go-to style. It's straightforward, without any tricky bits.

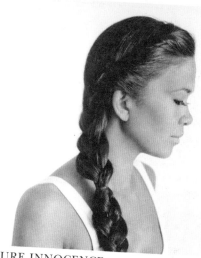

PURE INNOCENCE
If you don't have time for a full French braid, this style—which incorporates a twist—is the perfect solution.

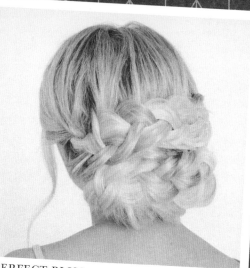

PERFECT BLISS
This is one of the fastest updos ever. All you have to do is create four basic braids to look elegant.

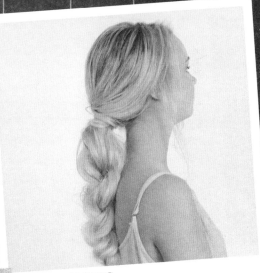

CATWALK CHIC
This perfectly textured braid allows you to work fast. Put your hair in a ponytail, make a basic braid, and you're all set.

winding
ROAD

*This updo, reminiscent of the Renaissance era, is given a messy bohemian twist. The **multiple braids** add a unique textural element, while the **ribbons intertwined** with the braids amp up the drama. No matter the occasion, this style is sure to wow everyone.*

difficulty
intermediate

minimum hair length
shoulder blades

what you'll need
hair clips
clear ponytail elastics (or a color that matches your hair)
clear small elastics (or a color that matches your hair)
6 yards (5.5m) ribbon
scissors
bobby pins
hairspray

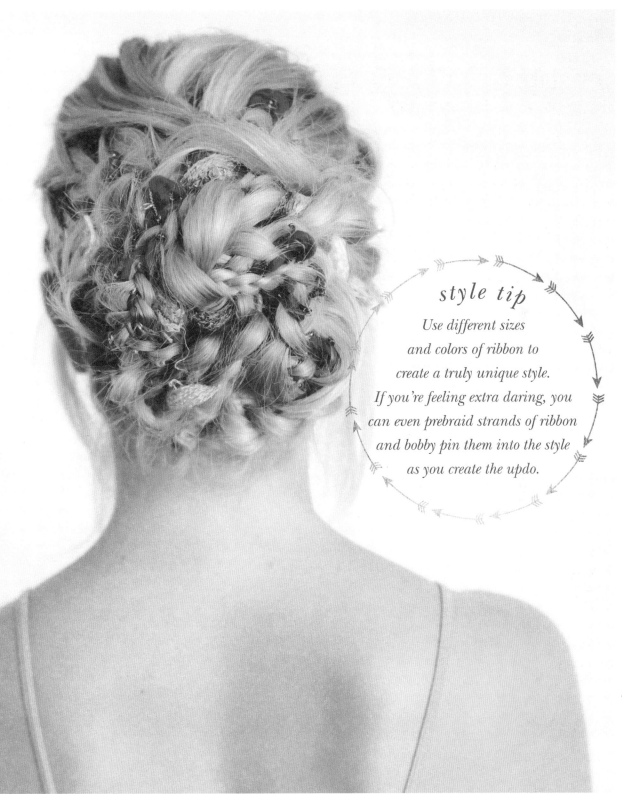

style tip

Use different sizes
and colors of ribbon to
create a truly unique style.
If you're feeling extra daring, you
can even prebraid strands of ribbon
and bobby pin them into the style
as you create the updo.

1 Section off and clip away the front of your hair from the back. Carve out a square section at the center of the back and secure with an elastic.

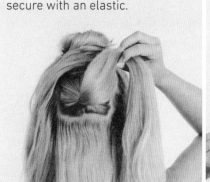

2 Cut a piece of ribbon twice the length of the ponytail. Slide it through the elastic until the ends are even.

Place the ribbon in the exterior sections

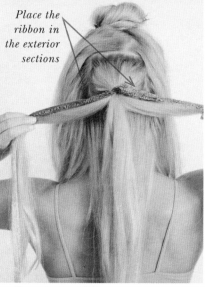

3 Divide the ponytail into three equal sections. Make a basic braid using the sections. Secure the end with an elastic.

This is the main braid

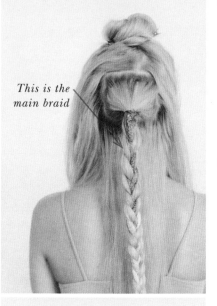

4 Place the remaining hair from the back into four ponytails. Cut four pieces of ribbon twice the length of each ponytail. Slide one through each elastic.

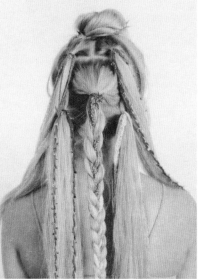

5 Divide each ponytail into three sections and basic braid them, starting with the ribbon in the exterior sections of each one. Secure each with an elastic.

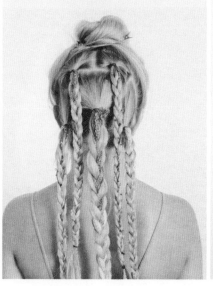

6 Release the clip from the front section and create a very loose basic braid (without ribbon) in the middle crown area. Secure with an elastic.

Make it low enough and wide enough to hide the elastics and parts beneath it

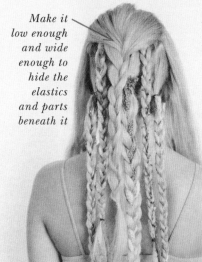

7 Create four more basic braids (without ribbon) using the remaining hair from the front section. You should have 10 braids total. Secure the ends of each braid with an elastic.

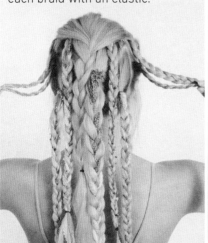

8 Pancake all of the braids. Adjust the ribbons so they are visible.

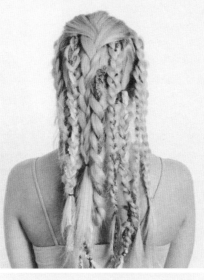

9 Clip away the three braids at the crown, exposing the main braid. Cross the four braids from the front sections over each other, above the main braid.

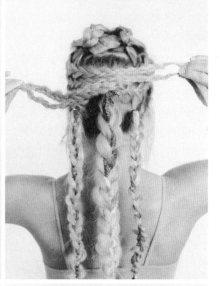

10 Secure the four braids with crisscrossed bobby pins.

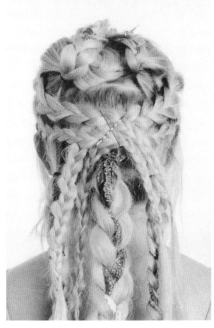

11 Gather all 10 braids together and wrap them loosely to form a bun.

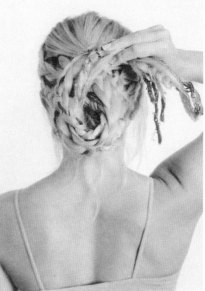

12 Secure the bun with bobby pins. Arrange the ribbons as desired so they are visible. Finish the style with hairspray.

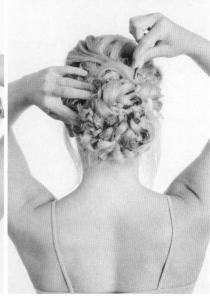

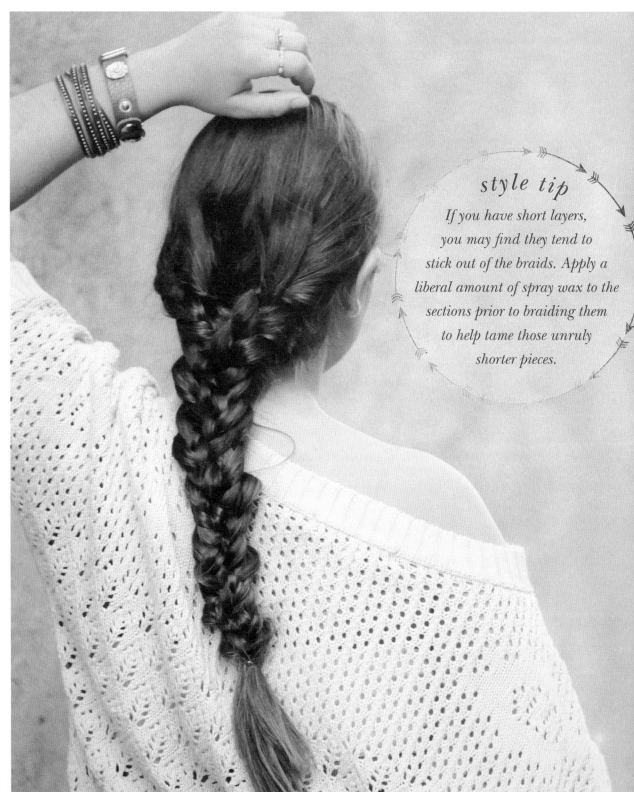

style tip

If you have short layers, you may find they tend to stick out of the braids. Apply a liberal amount of spray wax to the sections prior to braiding them to help tame those unruly shorter pieces.

tapestry

Weave your way to beautiful hair! This **lovely braid** has the appearance of an amazingly intricate piece of work. However, you only have to know how to do a basic **three-strand braid** in order to make it (though admirers need not know!).

difficulty
easy

minimum hair length
mid-back

what you'll need
hair clips
clear small elastics (or a color that matches your hair)
hairspray

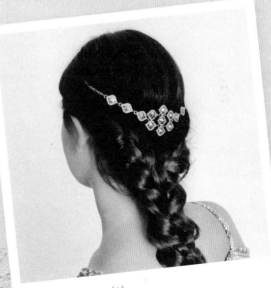

accessorize it!
Place the combs of a draping chain accessory near the front of your hair and allow the chains to hang down in the back to really highlight the woven texture.

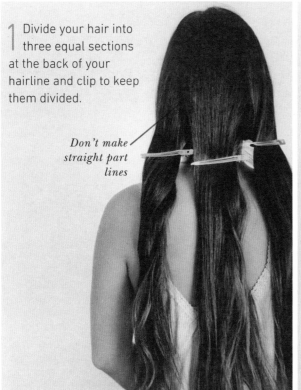

1 Divide your hair into three equal sections at the back of your hairline and clip to keep them divided.

Don't make straight part lines

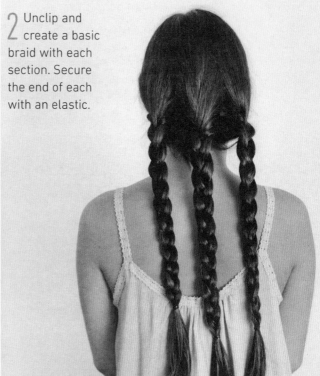

2 Unclip and create a basic braid with each section. Secure the end of each with an elastic.

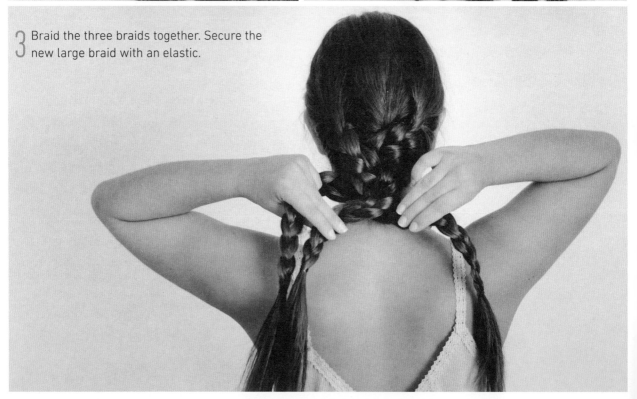

3 Braid the three braids together. Secure the new large braid with an elastic.

4 Pull on random loops to make the braid messier and more three-dimensional.

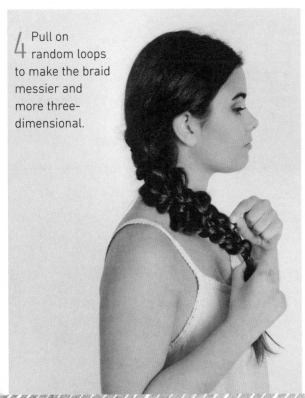

5 Cut or break the elastics from the original smaller braids, if they're visible. Finish the style with hairspray.

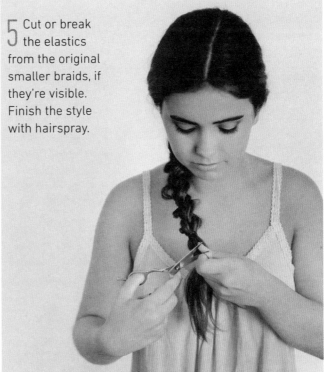

FINISHED LOOK

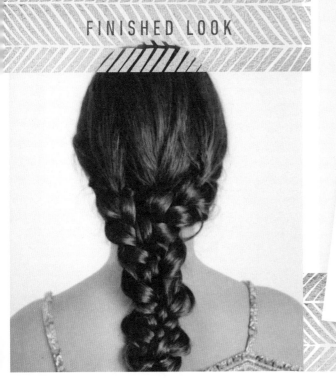

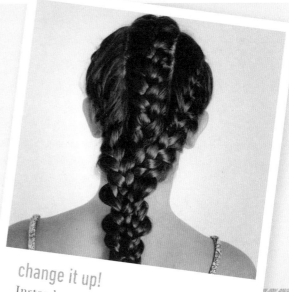

change it up!
Instead of basic breads, create three French braids and then braid them together at the bottom.

SOFT
rock

*If you want a punk rock look but are feeling a bit too lazy to put in a ton of effort, try this **twist on the traditional ponytail**. It can be done on freshly washed hair or on day-two unwashed hair with dry shampoo.*

difficulty
easy

minimum hair length
mid-back

what you'll need
large-barrel (1 ½ in.; 35mm) curling wand or iron
bobby pins
clear small elastics (or a color that matches your hair)
clear ponytail elastic (or a color that matches your hair)
teasing comb or brush
medium-barrel (1 in.; 19mm) curling wand or iron
hairspray

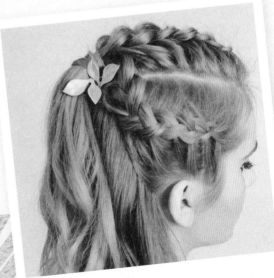

accessorize it!
Insert a pair of leaf pins near the base of the ponytail to complement the braids.

To look hard rock, try pumping up the volume by teasing the middle section before you braid to make it stand up more like a mohawk. Leave the sides unteased to keep them close to your head.

1 Using the large curling wand or iron, create beach waves all over your head.

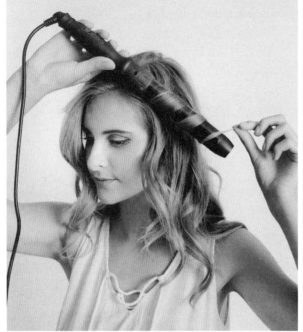

2 Split the top half of your hair into three sections, with the middle section about 3 inches (7.5cm) wide. Pin the sections out of the way.

The back part goes from the middle of one ear to the other

3 Dutch braid each section all the way to the ends. Secure each with an elastic.

Pancake the braids that remain against the scalp

4 Pull all three braids together into a high half-ponytail and secure with an elastic. Unbraid the sections below the elastic.

Break or cut the elastics rather than pulling them out

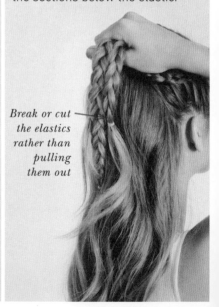

5 Tease the ponytail. Wrap the ponytail elastic with a section of hair from below the ponytail. Using the medium curling wand or iron, curl the ends of the ponytail and the ends of the loose hair. Finish the style with hairspray.

style tip

Place a bobby pin under the ponytail to secure the hair you wrapped the ponytail with.

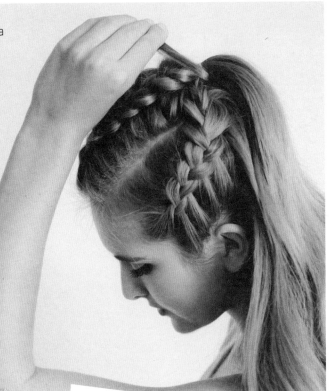

FINISHED LOOK

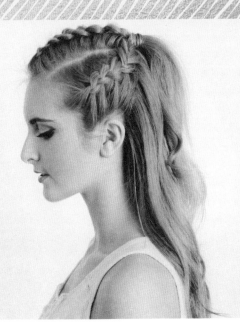

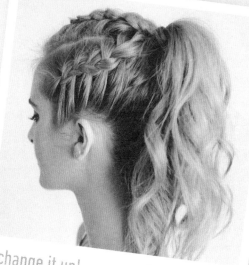

change it up!
Pull all of your hair up into the ponytail for an edgier look.

festival
PRINCESS

This romantic style is given an edgy flair with the addition of **pigtail buns.** *Wear it to a Renaissance fair, or take it to city streets—no matter where you go, others will marvel at your funky 'do. Achieve as much texture as you can to really make it shine!*

difficulty
easy

minimum hair length
top of shoulders

what you'll need
dry shampoo
large-barrel (1½ in.; 35mm) or larger curling wand or iron
teasing comb or brush
bobby pins
hairspray

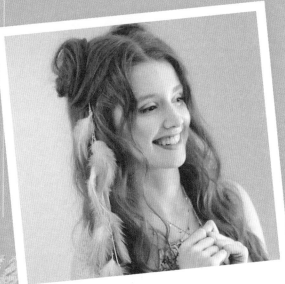

accessorize it!
Turn this style up a notch by attaching a feather clip-in extension under one of the buns.

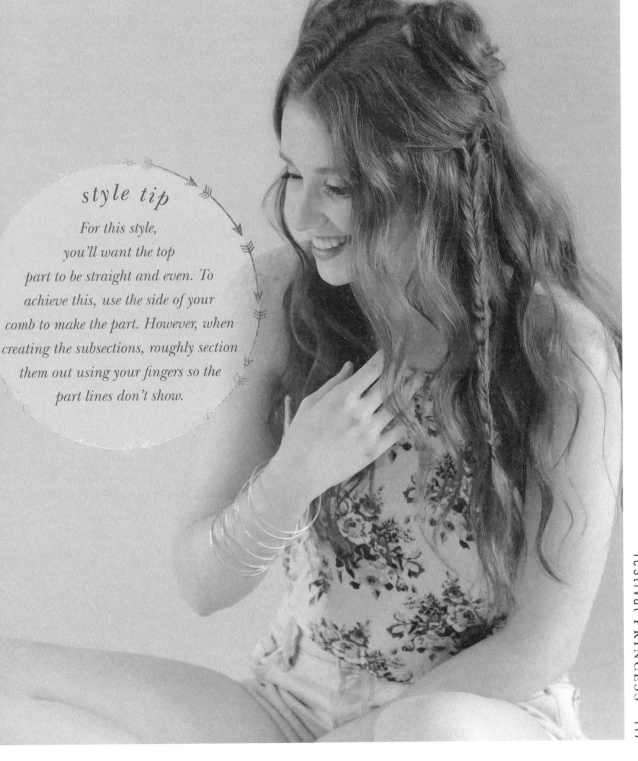

style tip

For this style, you'll want the top part to be straight and even. To achieve this, use the side of your comb to make the part. However, when creating the subsections, roughly section them out using your fingers so the part lines don't show.

1 Prep your roots with dry shampoo and create beach waves. Part your hair down the middle.

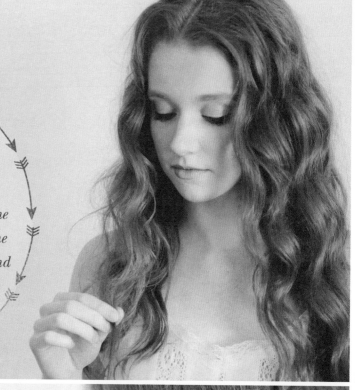

style tip

To add volume, hold the bottom of a curled strand. Next, use the index finger and thumb of your other hand to pinch the hair right above the hand holding the bottom of the hair. Pull your index and thumb lightly up and out along the strand to fan out the hair.

2 On either side of the part, tease 2 inches (5cm) of hair parallel to the part. Leave hair unteased around the hairline.

3 On each side of the part, use a section 2 inches (5cm) back from the hairline and make a small fishtail braid. Tease the ends to secure. Get messy as you pancake both braids.

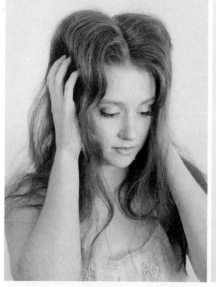

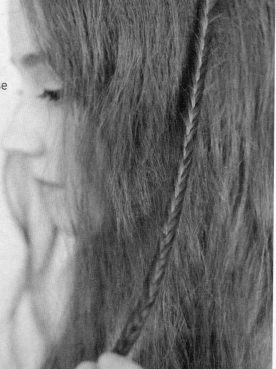

4 On each side of the part, make a loose, messy bun using the braid. Pin the buns on either side of your crown with bobby pins.

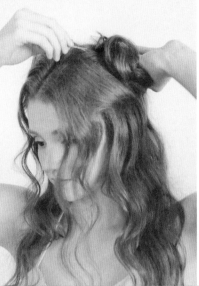

5 Pancake both braids to make them appear fuller.

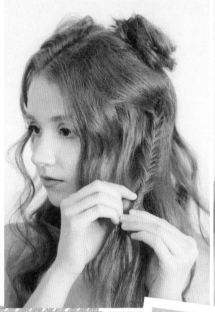

6 Finish the style with hairspray and scrunch the curls.

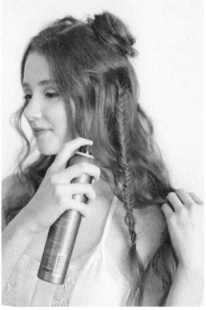

FINISHED LOOK

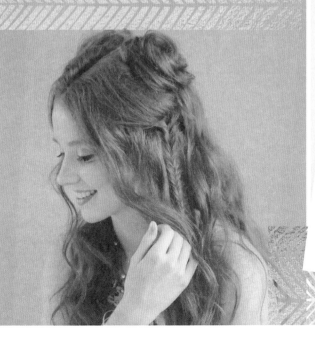

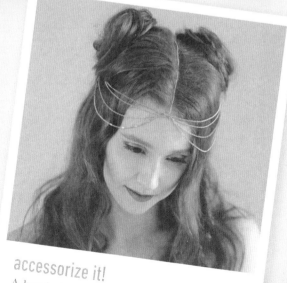

accessorize it!
A head chain can add a tribal vibe to the style.

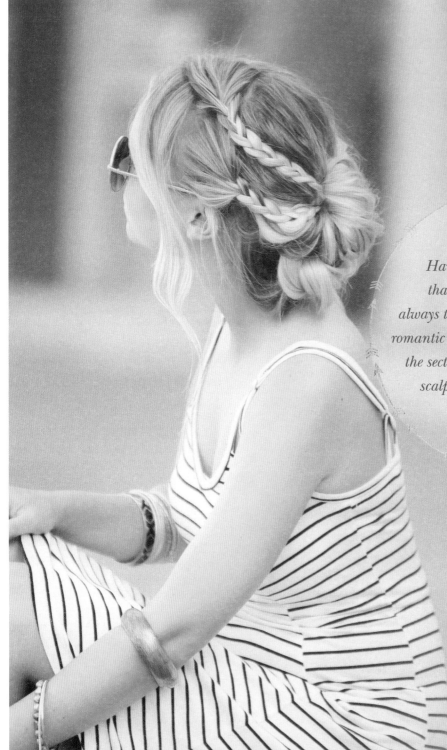

style tip

Having extreme part lines that show your scalp isn't always the best look, especially for a romantic boho style like this one. Keep the sections loose and low so your scalp doesn't show where the braids are parted.

GRACEFUL
beauty

This isn't your average bun updo. **Small braids, twists,** *and a* **topsy-tail** *come together to make a simple yet detailed look. You can show off your effortless style for anything from a casual day at the park to a dressy cocktail party.*

difficulty
easy

minimum hair length
shoulder blades

what you'll need
clear small elastics (or a color that matches your hair)
clear ponytail elastic (or a color that matches your hair)
bobby pins
hairspray

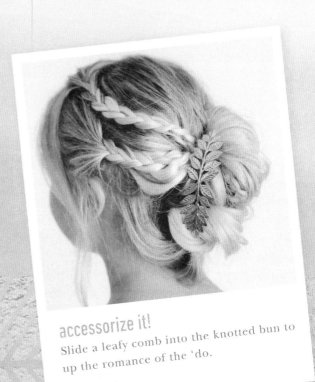

accessorize it!
Slide a leafy comb into the knotted bun to up the romance of the 'do.

1 Create four small basic braids along your front hairline and secure each with an elastic.

2 Section the hair from ear to ear across the back. Place the hair above the part, including the braids, into a loose ponytail. Leave the hair below it down.

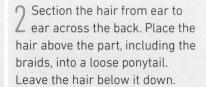

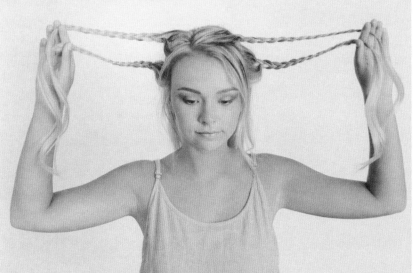

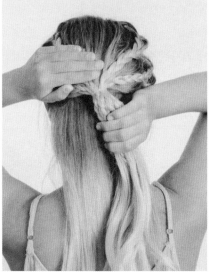

3 Make a hole with your finger above the ponytail and flip the ponytail up and through the hole.

This is called a topsy-tail

4 Take your hair, including the ponytail, and twist it around twice.

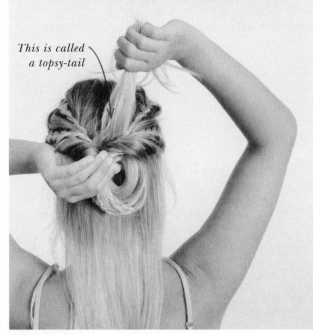

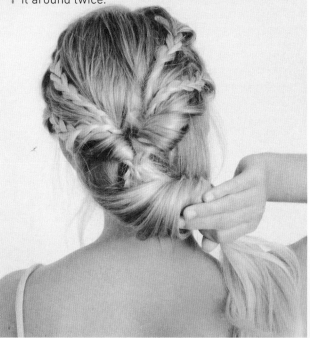

5 Place the twisted hair through the hole above the ponytail. This will create a vertical loop at the nape.

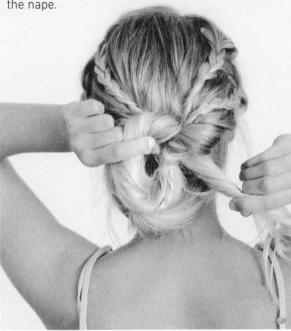

6 Twist the tail once and bring it across the loop.

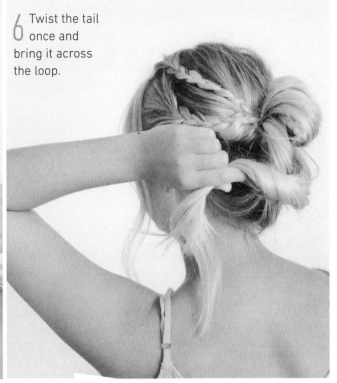

7 Tuck the tail through the loop at the nape, forming a knotted bun. Pin the entire knotted bun, loosening as needed. Finish the style with hairspray.

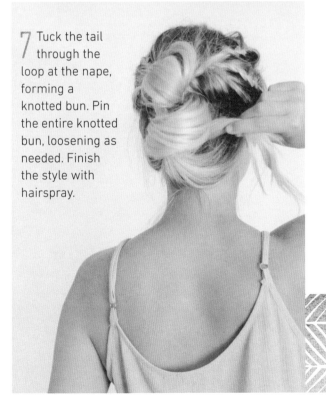

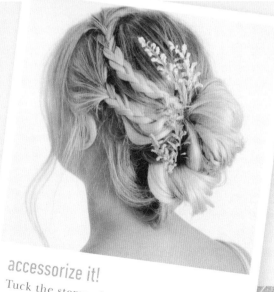

accessorize it!
Tuck the stems of some floral sprigs into one side of the knotted bun, making sure they stick out from the hairstyle.

ROMANTIC
soul

*Capture the look of a starry-eyed romantic with this **braided headband** style. Whether your hair is naturally curly, wavy, or straight, this look will make you feel like you've stepped out of a wonderful dream.*

difficulty
easy

minimum hair length
shoulder blades

what you'll need
large-barrel (1½ in.; 35mm) curling wand or iron
hair clips
one-clip clip-in extensions (optional)
clear small elastics (or a color that matches your hair)
bobby pins
hairspray

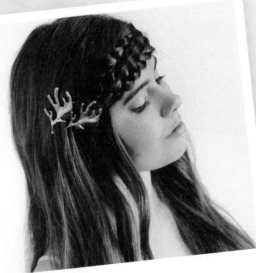

accessorize it!
Use an ornate clip-in right under one of the braids to add some drama.

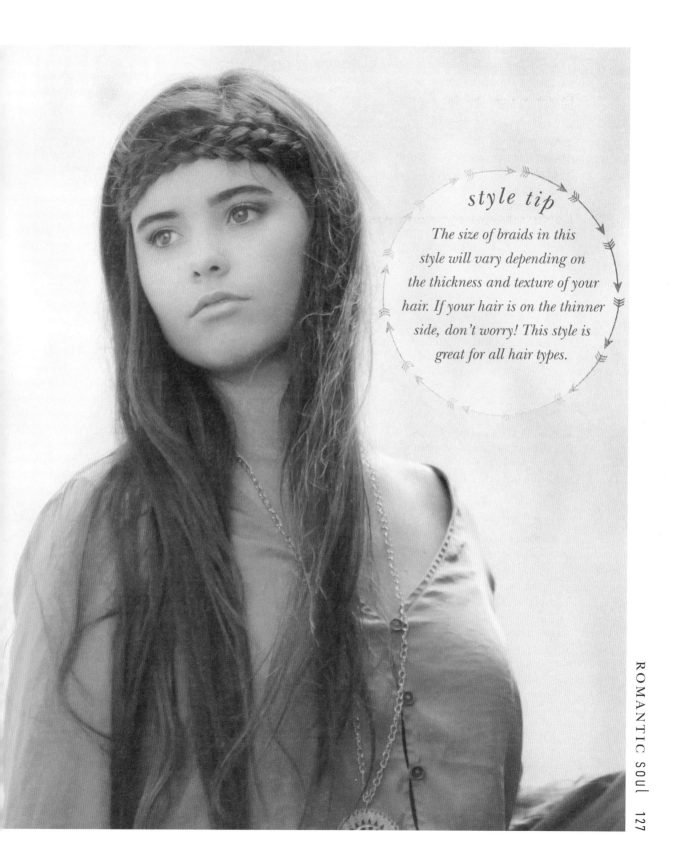

style tip

The size of braids in this
style will vary depending on
the thickness and texture of your
hair. If your hair is on the thinner
side, don't worry! This style is
great for all hair types.

1 Create beach waves. Section off the top crown area and clip it away.

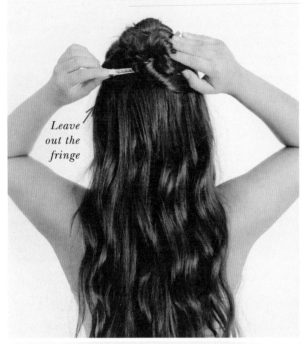

Leave out the fringe

2 Make a section 2 inches (5cm) wide above each ear. (If your hair is thin, add a one-clip hair extension to each section.)

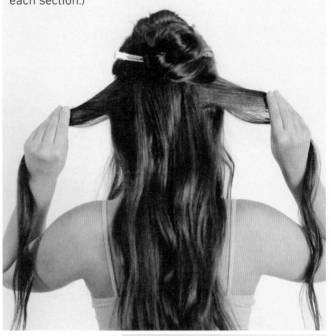

3 Create a basic braid with each section and secure each with an elastic.

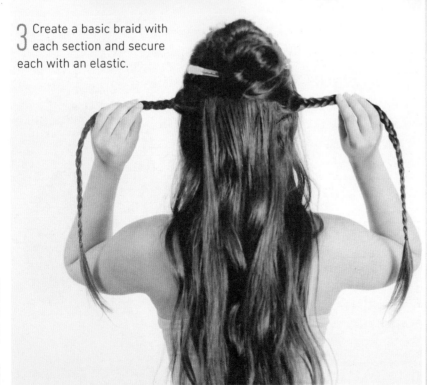

4 Pancake the braids to make them appear fuller.

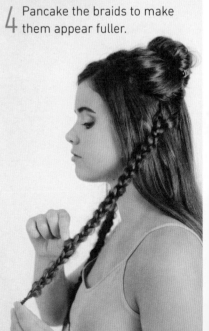

5 Wrap the braids across your forehead. Hide and secure the tails of the braids with bobby pins.

Bobby pin the tail directly into the braid

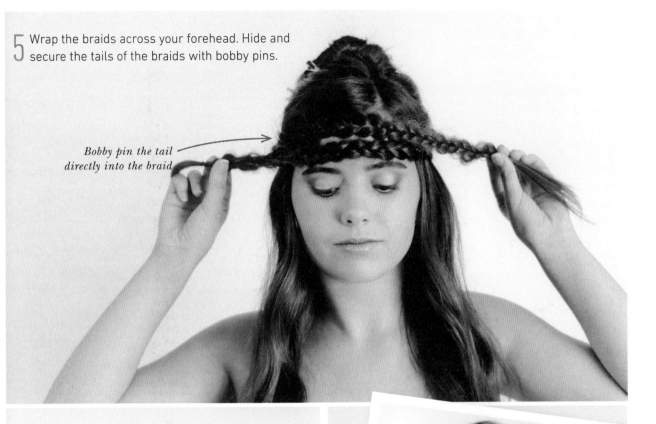

6 Remove the hair clip and make sure the bases of the braids are covered with the loose hair. Finish the style with hairspray.

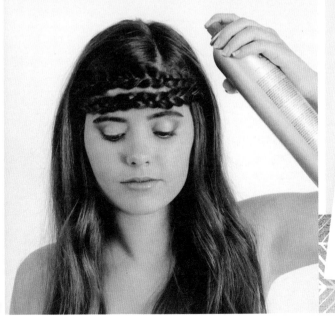

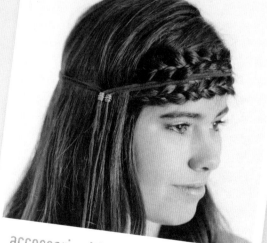

accessorize it!

For an extra dose of hippie chic, wrap faux leather ribbons around your head and on top of the braids. You can tie the ends into a simple knot on the side.

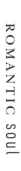

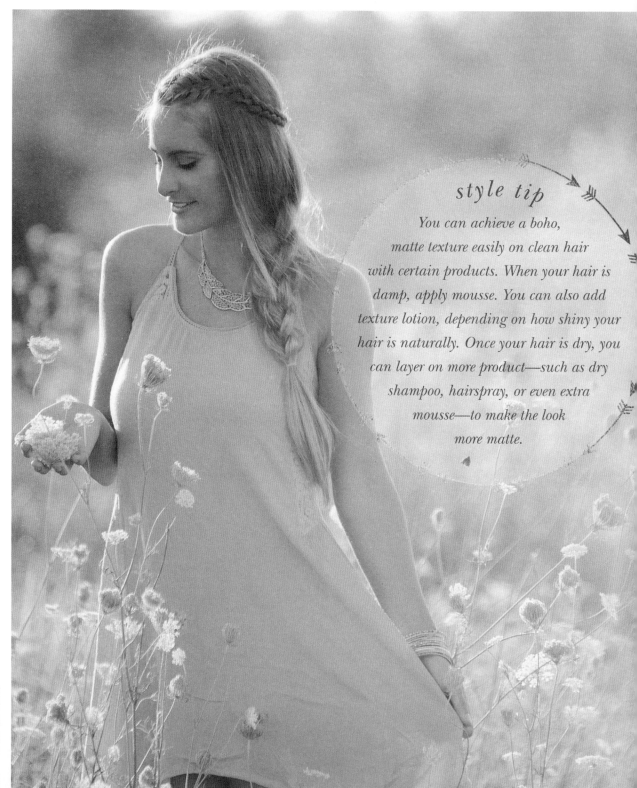

You can achieve a boho, matte texture easily on clean hair with certain products. When your hair is damp, apply mousse. You can also add texture lotion, depending on how shiny your hair is naturally. Once your hair is dry, you can layer on more product—such as dry shampoo, hairspray, or even extra mousse—to make the look more matte.

WANDERING
belle

*Look chic while you're on the go! This **beautiful braid** works for any destination and climate your travel-ready heart desires. The best part: it's an ideal way to wear your hair when it hasn't been freshly washed.*

difficulty
easy

minimum hair length
mid-back

what you'll need
comb or brush
bobby pin
clear small elastics (or a color that matches your hair)

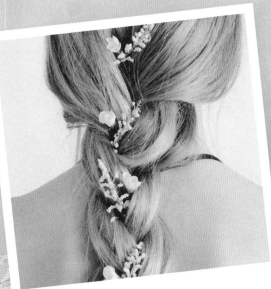

accessorize it!
Tuck flowers into the lower braid to add some whimsy.

1 Part your hair down the middle.

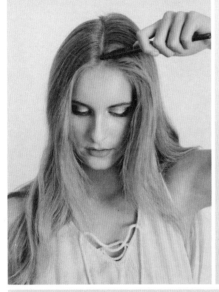

2 Beginning at the top on one side of your head, Dutch braid your hair, adding in hair only from the top section as you go.

Pancake as you braid

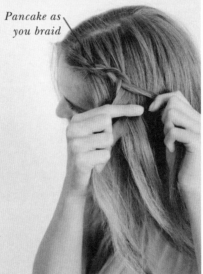

3 Once you're about 1 inch (2.5cm) past your ear, stop adding in hair and create a basic braid to the ends. Secure with a bobby pin.

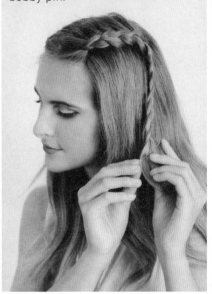

4 Repeat steps 2 and 3 on the other side. Pancake both braids.

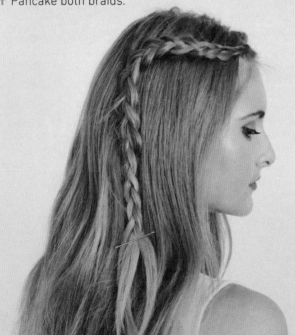

5 Join the braids in the center at the back of your head with an elastic.

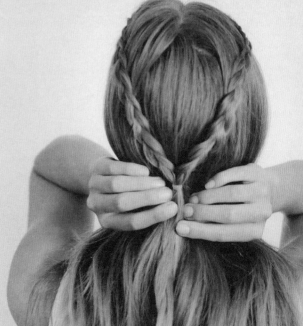

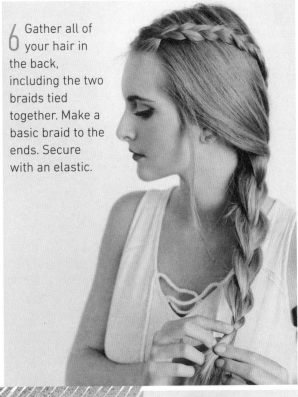

6 Gather all of your hair in the back, including the two braids tied together. Make a basic braid to the ends. Secure with an elastic.

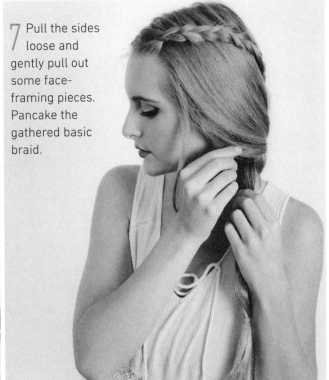

7 Pull the sides loose and gently pull out some face-framing pieces. Pancake the gathered basic braid.

FINISHED
LOOK

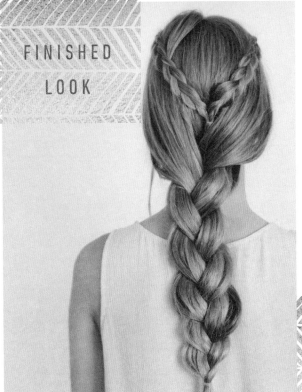

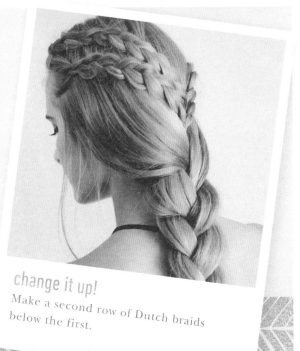

change it up!
Make a second row of Dutch braids below the first.

BUTTERFLY
effect

*Whether you want to be stylish at the gym or just hang out with friends, this **rippling braided half-updo** is the perfect casual look. While it has the appearance of a **fishtail**, it's actually a **basic braid pancaked wide**—a simple concept that's very easy to construct.*

difficulty
easy

minimum hair length
shoulder blades

what you'll need
clear small elastics (or a color that matches your hair)
hairspray

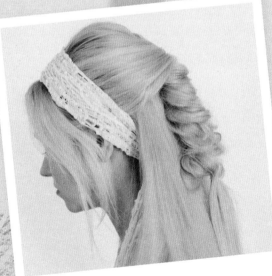

accessorize it!
You will look like an artist's muse with a fringed, extra-long lacy scarf tied around your head.

style tip

If you have shorter layers, you may consider doing the variation of this style. It would provide additional security in the middle for those layers that want to pop out of the braid.

1 Beginning with straight hair, section out the front half of your hair and create a basic braid. Secure the end of the braid with an elastic.

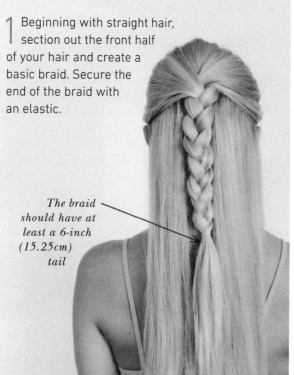

The braid should have at least a 6-inch (15.25cm) tail

2 Starting from the bottom near the elastic band, pancake the braid.

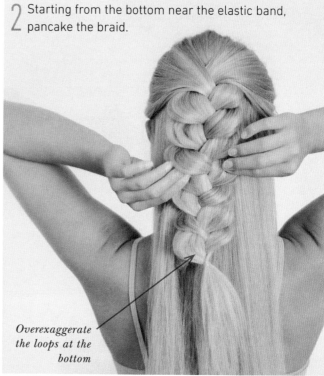

Overexaggerate the loops at the bottom

3 Take a very small piece from the edge of each loop and gently loosen it further. Finish the style with hairspray.

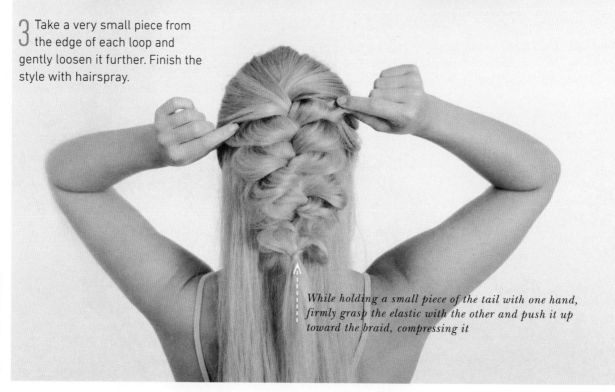

While holding a small piece of the tail with one hand, firmly grasp the elastic with the other and push it up toward the braid, compressing it

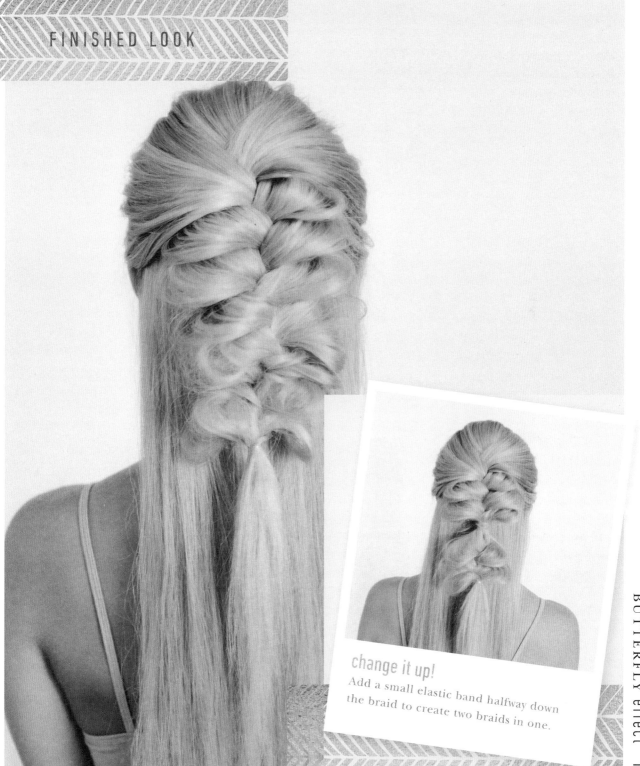

change it up!

Add a small elastic band halfway down the braid to create two braids in one.

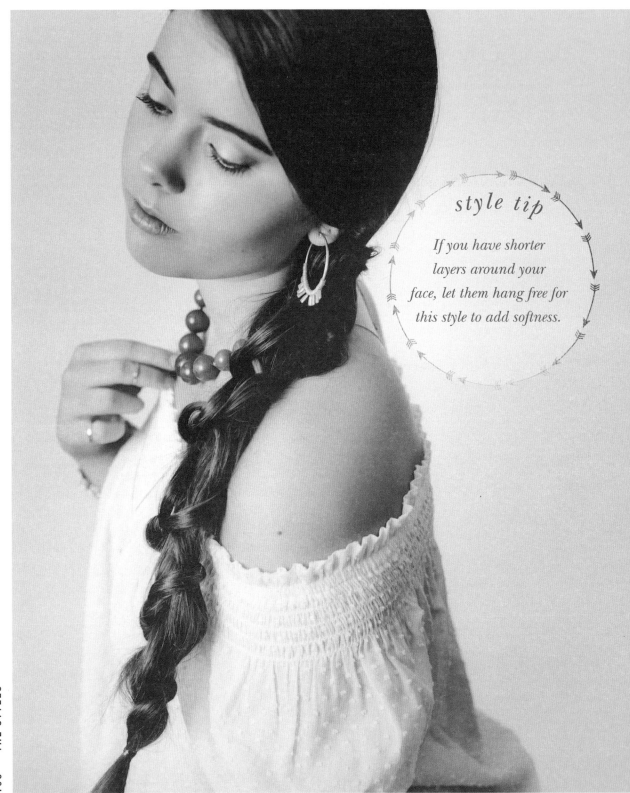

style tip

If you have shorter layers around your face, let them hang free for this style to add softness.

DELICATE
thread

Add some refinement to the average side pony with this style. Using a **chain-link technique,** *you can wrap your ponytail in gentle laces of hair. This graceful style pairs perfectly with a gentle, flowing dress for a look that's very romantic.*

difficulty
intermediate

minimum hair length
shoulder blades

what you'll need
hair clip (optional)
clear ponytail elastic (or a color that matches your hair)
bobby pins
clear small elastic (or a color that matches your hair)
hairspray

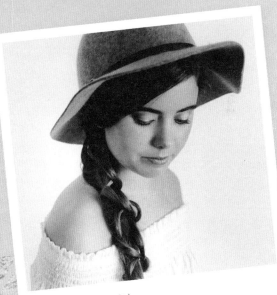

accessorize it!
Because this style sits low on your neck, a hat is a wonderful accessory that lends a flirty vibe.

1 Starting with straight hair, section out a 1-inch (2.5cm) square section at the right side of your back hairline.

2 Gather the rest of your hair into a low ponytail right above the 1-inch (2.5cm) square section. Secure at the top with an elastic.

3 Split the section into two pieces. Wrap them around the ponytail and tie them together at the front of the elastic. Secure with a bobby pin at the top of the tie.

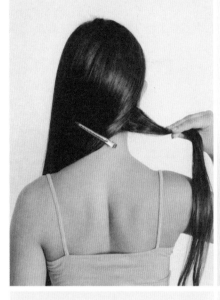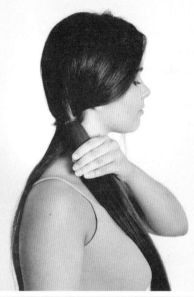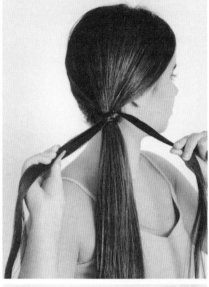

4 Tie the pieces again at the front of the ponytail 1 inch (2.5cm) down from the elastic.

5 Bring the two pieces to the back of the ponytail and tie them together 1 inch (2.5cm) down from the previous tie.

6 Bring the two pieces to the front of the ponytail and tie them together 1 inch (2.5cm) down from the previous tie.

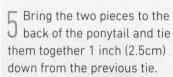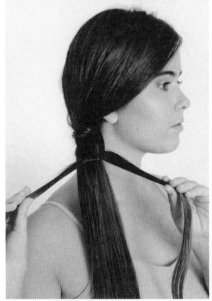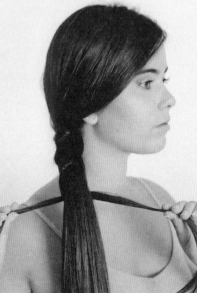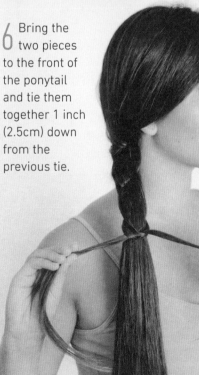

7 Take two small pieces from the back of the ponytail and add them to the original two pieces.

Twist the new pieces with the old pieces

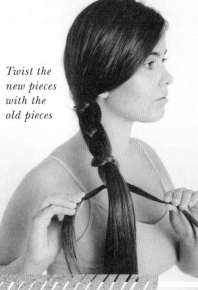

8 Continue wrapping and tying the two pieces until you get to the bottom. Secure with an elastic.

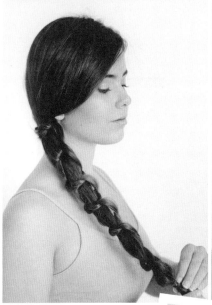

9 Pancake the chains. Place a bobby pin through any tied areas that appear to be loose. Finish the style with hairspray.

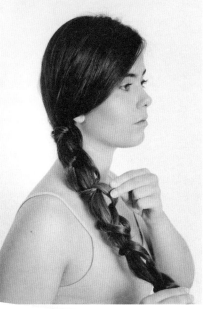

FINISHED LOOK

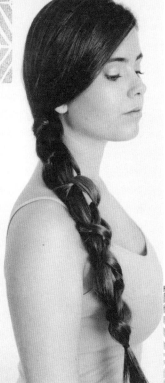

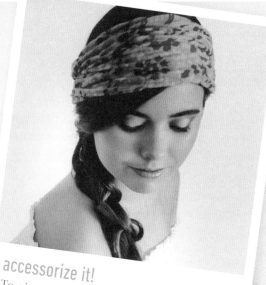

accessorize it!
To give your look a cute, casual feel, place a headband around your head and let it sit just above the low ponytail.

DAISY
chain

Crown braids don't always have to be big and full. This hairstyle uses *four chain-link-style braids* to create a unique, piece-y look. Dress it down for a trip to the coffee shop, or dress it up to impress party guests with your runway-ready hair.

difficulty
intermediate

minimum hair length
mid-back

what you'll need
hair clips
clear small elastics (or a color that matches your hair)
bobby pins
hairspray

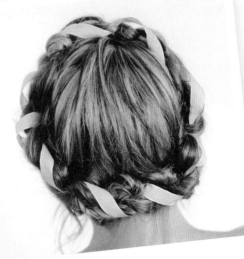

accessorize it!
To soften your look, weave ribbon through the chain links.

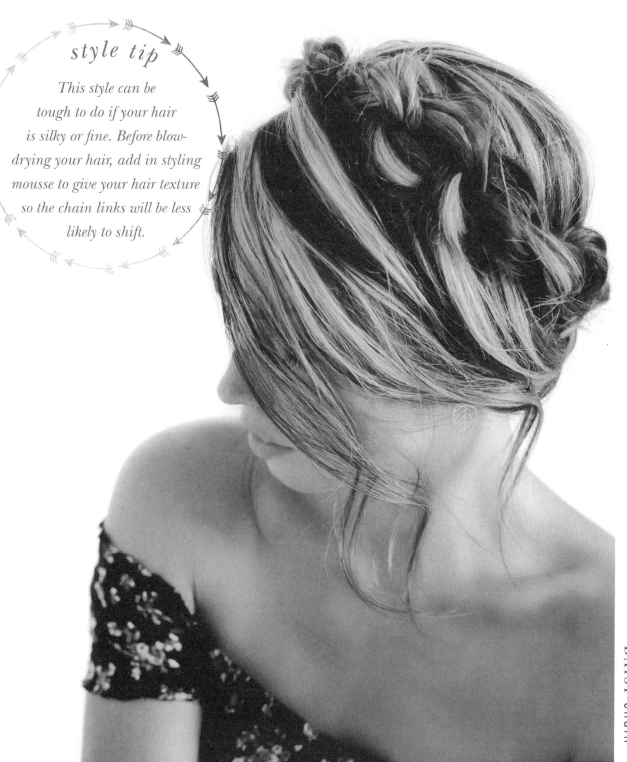

style tip

This style can be
tough to do if your hair
is silky or fine. Before blow-
drying your hair, add in styling
mousse to give your hair texture
so the chain links will be less
likely to shift.

1 Split your hair into four sections—two side sections and two sections in the back—without creating part lines. Clip them away.

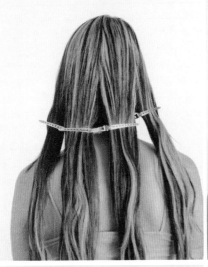

2 Starting with the right-side section, split it into two smaller sections and tie them together.

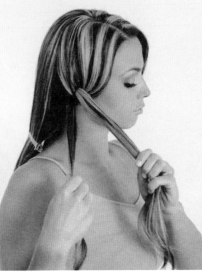

3 Continue tying the section over and over, leaving 1 inch (2.5cm) between each tie, until you reach the end.

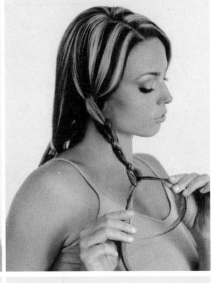

4 Secure the end of the chain-link braid with an elastic.

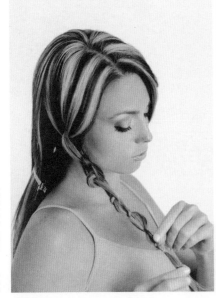

5 Repeat steps 2 through 4 on the remaining three sections.

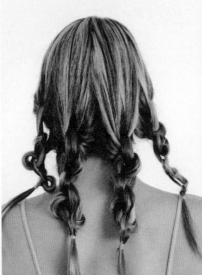

6 Take the two back sections and place them up and around the top of your head like a headband.

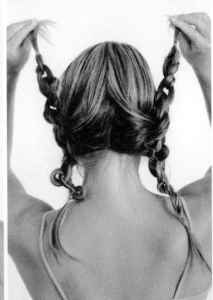

THE STYLES

7 Tie the ends together while hiding the elastics. Secure with bobby pins.

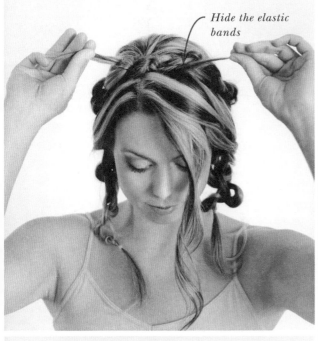

Hide the elastic bands

8 Take the two side sections and wrap them around the back. Tie the ends together and secure with bobby pins.

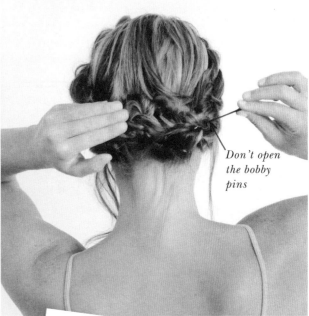

Don't open the bobby pins

9 Loosen the individual chain links and secure them with bobby pins. Finish the style with hairspray.

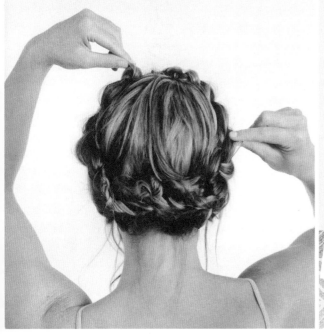

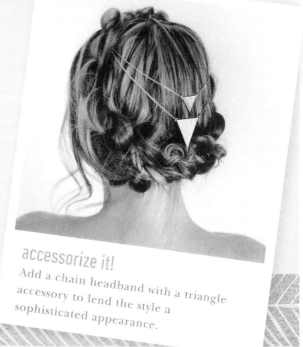

accessorize it!
Add a chain headband with a triangle accessory to lend the style a sophisticated appearance.

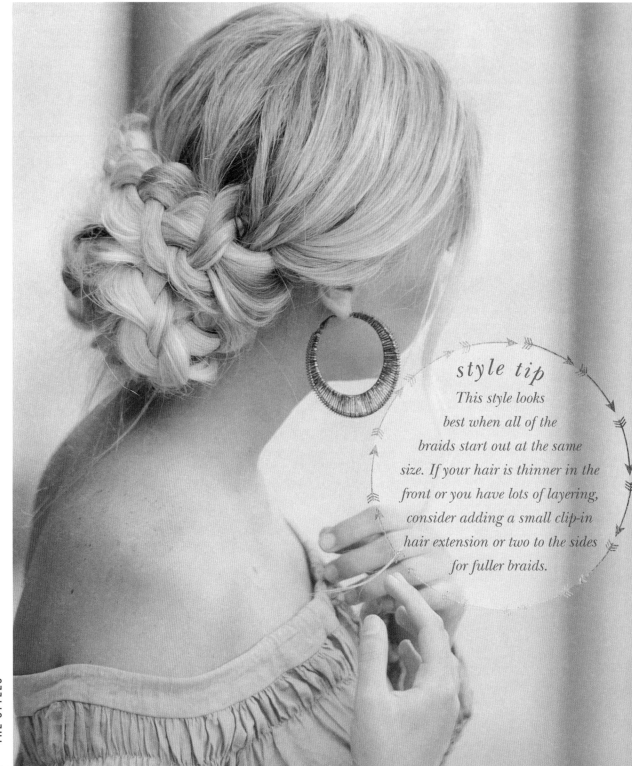

style tip

This style looks best when all of the braids start out at the same size. If your hair is thinner in the front or you have lots of layering, consider adding a small clip-in hair extension or two to the sides for fuller braids.

PERFECT
bliss

This **braided updo** might be on the list of easiest updos ever. Using **four regular basic braids,** you will be able to create a full, textured style. Embrace the simple pleasure of everything coming together just like you want it to.

minimum hair length
shoulder blades

what you'll need
hair clips
clear ponytail elastics (or a color that matches your hair)
clear small elastics (or a color that matches your hair)
bobby pins
hairspray

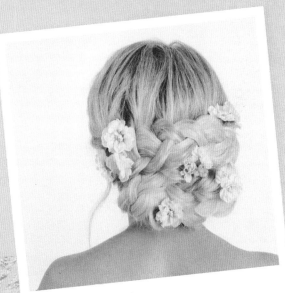

accessorize it!
Randomly pin small flowers throughout the back of this braided updo for a truly delicate touch.

1 Split your hair into four sections—two side sections and two sections in the back—without creating part lines. Place the two back sections into low ponytails using elastics.

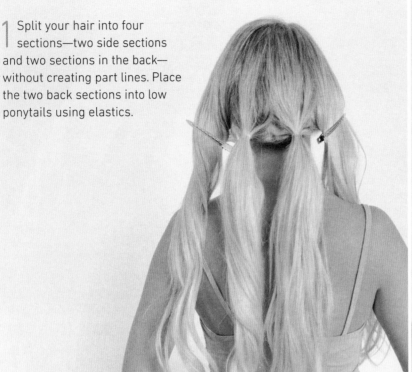

2 Create a basic braid for each of the four sections, and secure the ends with elastics.

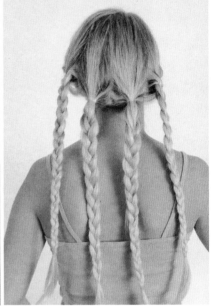

3 Loosen each braid and the crown area.

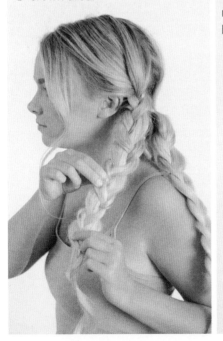

4 Wrap, lay, and bobby pin the two back sections near the nape of your neck to simulate a bun while hiding the elastics.

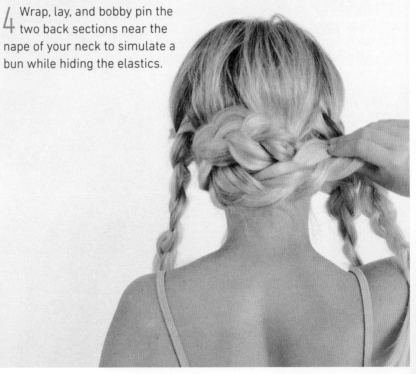

5 Bring the side sections to the back, laying them across the top of the bun. Bobby pin the braids. Finish the style with hairspray.

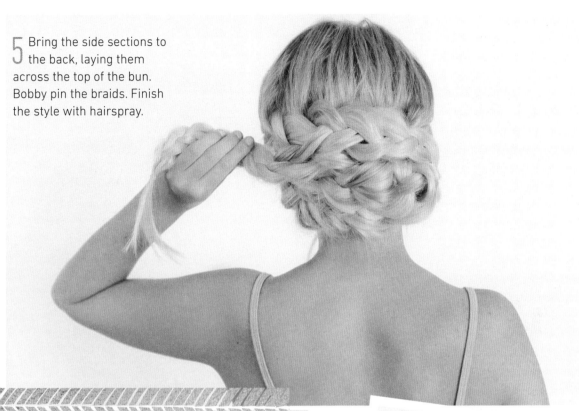

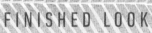

FINISHED LOOK

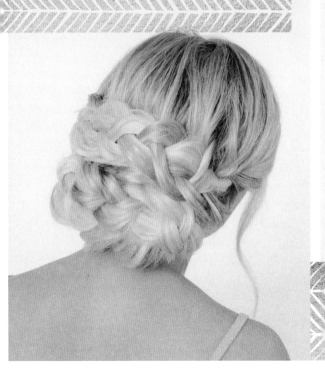

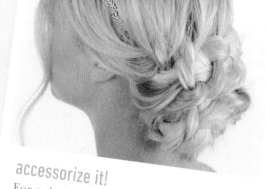

accessorize it!
For a dash of elegance, slide in a simple leafy gold headband to finish off this textured updo.

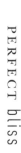

6 STYLES FOR SHOULDER-LENGTH HAIR

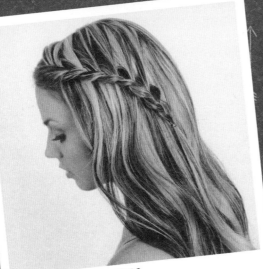

GENTLE WATERFALL
The great thing about waterfall braids is they don't require long hair, especially if you keep the braid high.

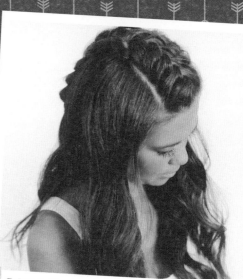

BOHO PUNK
This simple mowhawk braid can be done on almost any hair and looks extra cute on shoulder-length hair.

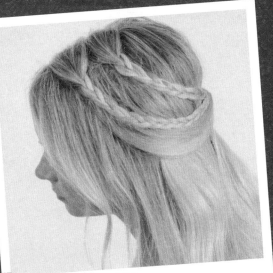

WHIMSICAL ROOTS
Although your braids will need to be pulled tighter to reach the back, this style looks amazing when complete.

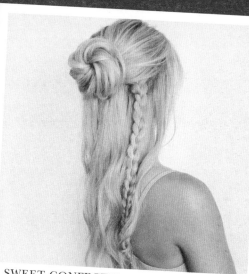

SWEET CONFECTION
This style is a no-brainer for shoulder-length hair. Combining a bun and braid, you get a unique, multitextured style.

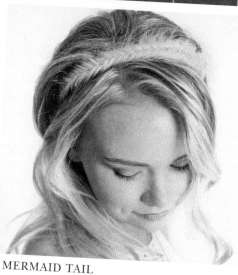

MERMAID TAIL
This fishtail crown is created using hair extensions, so it can be done on even the shortest of styles.

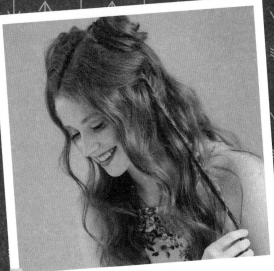

FESTIVAL PRINCESS
A half-up bun is always a crowd-pleaser for shorter hair—and when you have two, it's even better!

SMOOTH
grooves

*This take on a **half-up style** includes a **lace Dutch braid** curved around the back. Though it's a more difficult style to put together, it works for any occasion, so give it a go whenever you have the time.*

difficulty
challenging

minimum hair length
shoulder blades

what you'll need
large-barrel (1½ in.; 35mm) curling wand or iron
clear small elastics (or a color that matches your hair)
hairspray

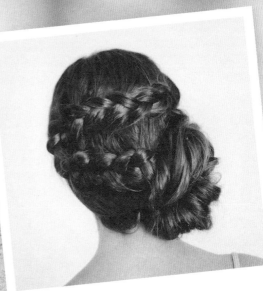

change it up!
Wrap the loose hair into a side bun below your right ear.

If your hair is thinner toward the top, consider adding a clip-in hair extension at the crown. This will serve as the hair to be included in the braid, creating a fuller look.

1 Create beach waves. Take a chunk of hair from the right side as if you're beginning a Dutch braid.

2 Begin braiding sideways across the back. However, instead of adding hair to both sides of the braid, only add to the top side. This will create a lace braid.

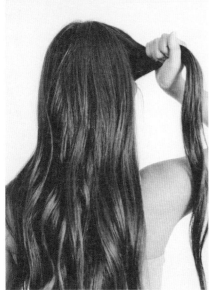

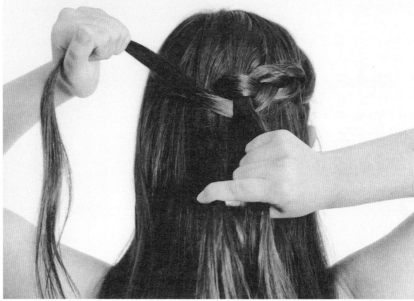

3 When you get to the left side, start curving the braid to change direction.

4 Once the braid is looped around, start adding hair to the top side again from under the main braid.

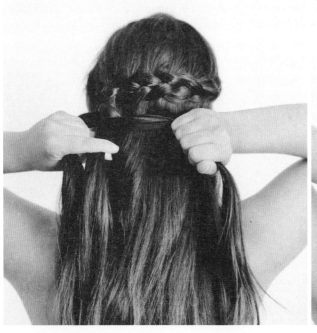

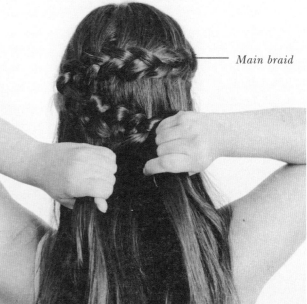

Main braid

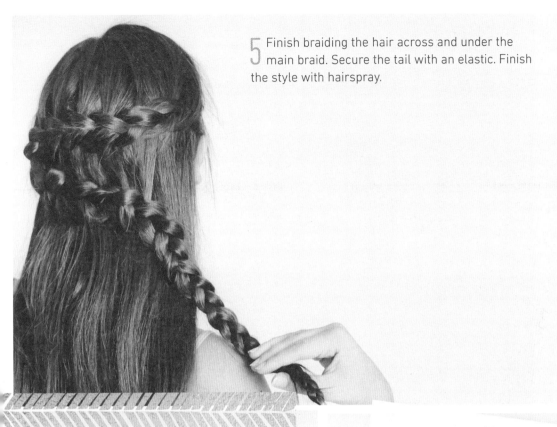

5 Finish braiding the hair across and under the main braid. Secure the tail with an elastic. Finish the style with hairspray.

FINISHED LOOK

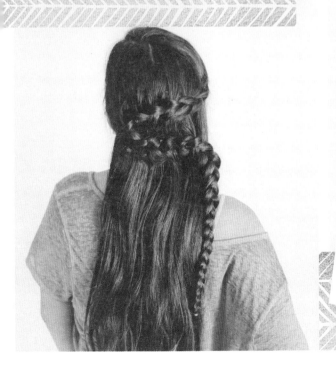

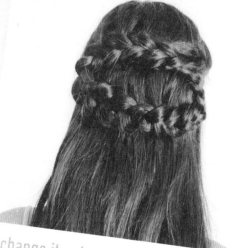

change it up!
Wrap and tuck the tail under the main braid and secure with bobby pins.

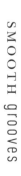

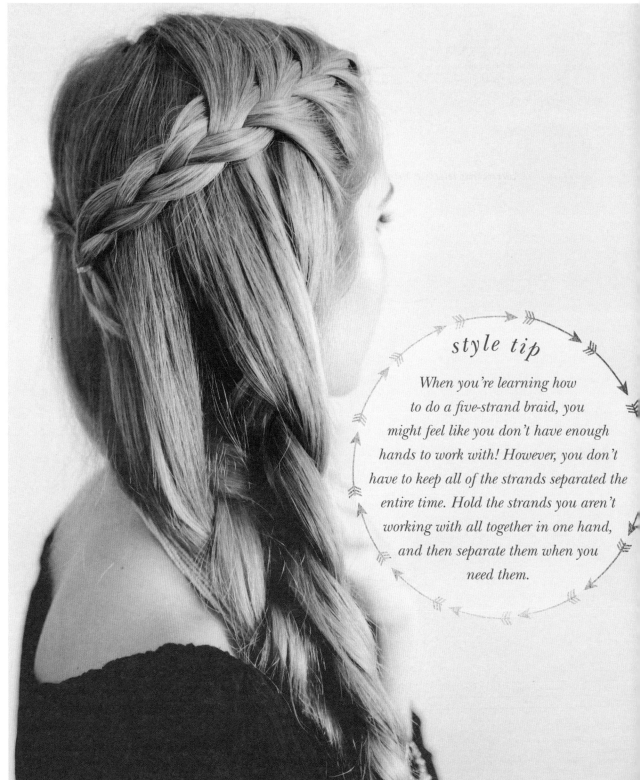

style tip

When you're learning how to do a five-strand braid, you might feel like you don't have enough hands to work with! However, you don't have to keep all of the strands separated the entire time. Hold the strands you aren't working with all together in one hand, and then separate them when you need them.

FLAMING
heart

*If you're wanting a little more of a braiding challenge, try out this **five-strand braid**. This style is done over your shoulder, allowing you to create it more easily. What results is a **loose, dreamy look** others will desire to imitate.*

difficulty
challenging

minimum hair length
mid-back

what you'll need
dry shampoo (optional)
comb
clear small elastics (or a color that matches your hair)
bobby pin (optional)
hairspray

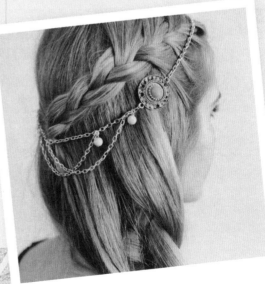

accessorize it!
Wear a hair chain to enhance the style's dreamy quality.

1 Use dry shampoo to add texture, if desired. Part your hair deep to one side.

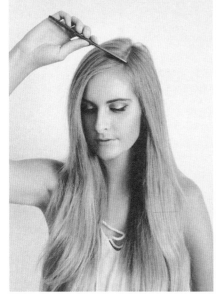

2 Working on the heavy side of your part, French braid from your part to just behind your ear. Next, create a basic braid to the ends.

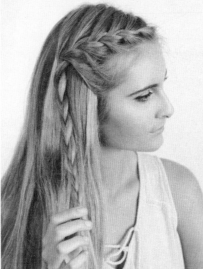

3 Take a section from the opposite side of your head, twist it upward, and join it with the first braid behind your head using an elastic.

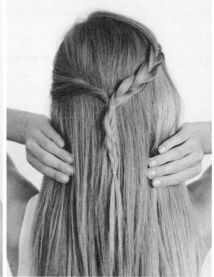

4 Gather your hair over one shoulder and, including the braid, divide it into five equal parts.

Add a bobby pin to keep the braid and twist secure, if needed

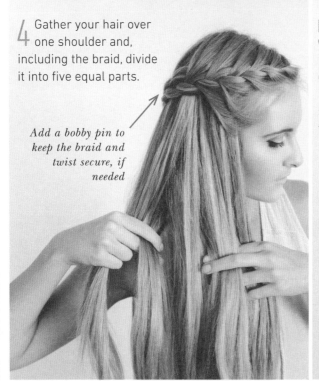

5 Take the rightmost section and cross it under the section directly to the left of it, and then over the section to the left of that one.

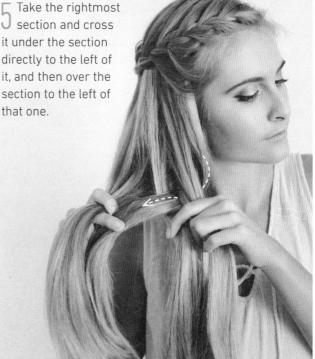

6 Switching to the left side of the braid, cross the leftmost section under the section directly to the right of it, and then over the section to the right of that one.

The pattern is: under, over, switch sides, under, over

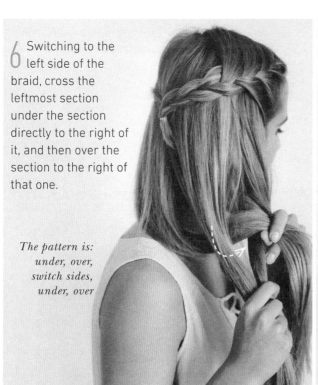

7 Repeat steps 5 and 6 until you reach the ends of your hair. Secure with an elastic. Finish the style with hairspray.

Gently pancake the outer sections, if desired

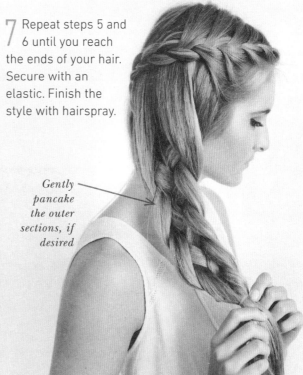

FINISHED LOOK

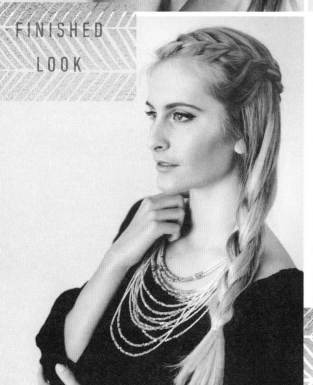

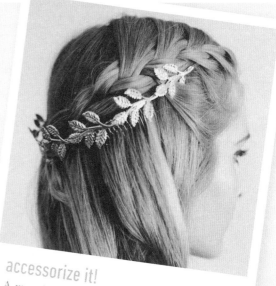

accessorize it!

A metal leaf headband, worn sideways rather than upright, accentuates the braid beneath it.

MANE
squeeze

*If you can put your hair into a ponytail, you can put together this style. This **loose bubble ponytail** adds a fun, flirty twist that goes against the norm. Rock this look on a casual day out with friends.*

minimum hair length
mid-back

what you'll need
clear ponytail elastics (or a color that matches your hair)
bobby pins
teasing comb
hairspray

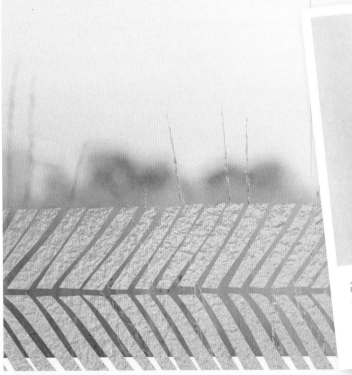
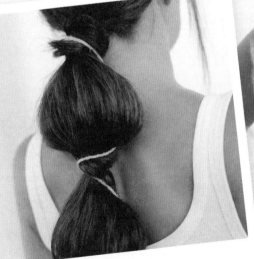

accessorize it!
Instead of wrapping hair around each elastic, use colored yarn or leather straps to play up the fun nature of the style.

1 Starting with straight hair, secure your hair into a low ponytail with an elastic, leaving out a few layers around your face.

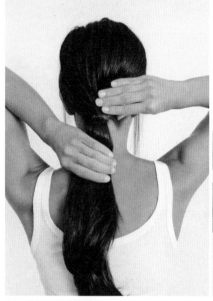

2 Take two skinny but long pieces of hair from the underside of the ponytail.

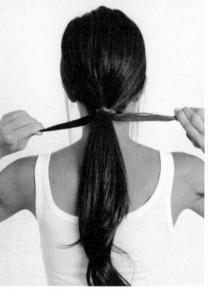

3 Wrap the two pieces around the elastic and tie them once on top of it.

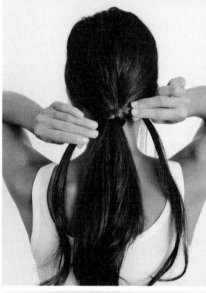

4 Slide two bobby pins into the crossover area, connecting them to the elastic.

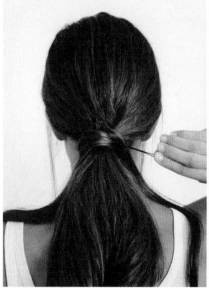

5 Leaving out the skinny pieces, tease the base of the ponytail. Place an elastic 3 inches (7.5cm) down from the previous one.

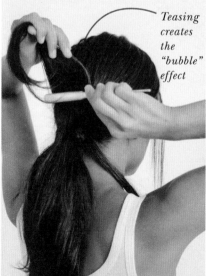

Teasing creates the "bubble" effect

6 Take the skinny pieces and cross them underneath the bubble. Bring them to the top and tie them around the elastic.

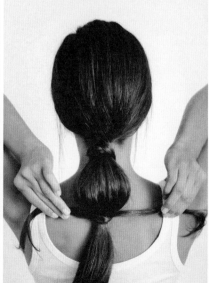

7 Loop the elastic around the ponytail to secure the small pieces. Repeat steps 2 through 7 until the last "bubble" is 3 inches (7.5cm) from the bottom.

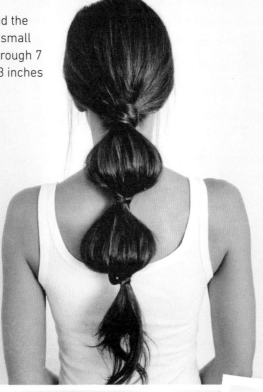

8 Loosen each tie to create more texture. Finish the style with hairspray.

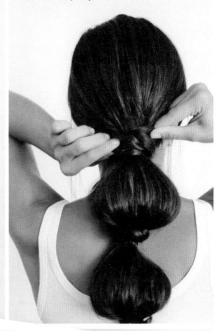

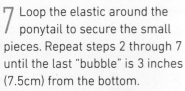

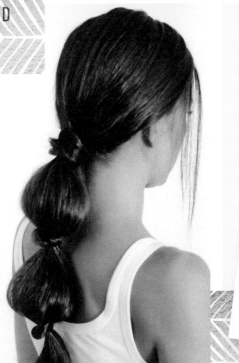

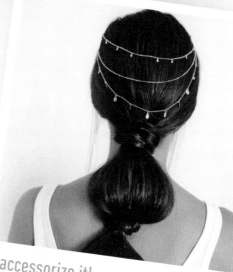

accessorize it!
A chain accessory can take this hairstyle from casual to dressy.

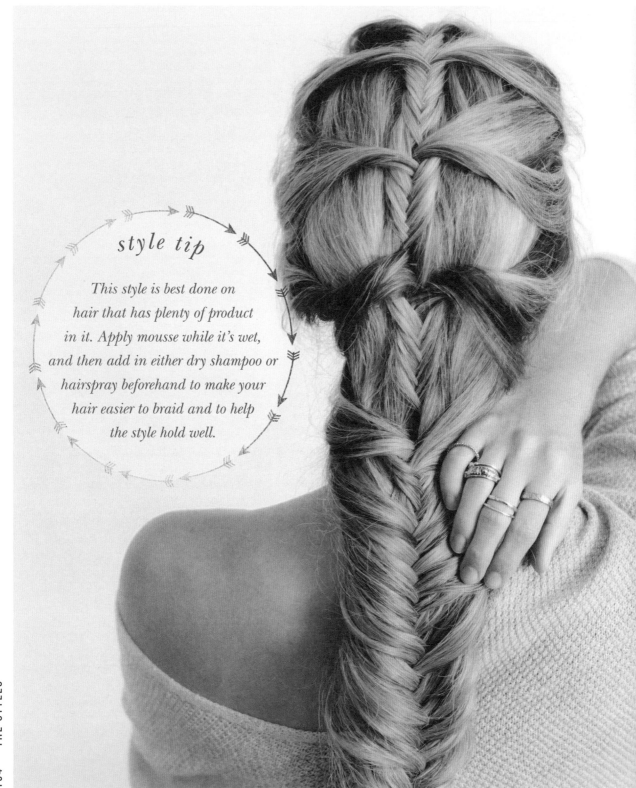

style tip

This style is best done on hair that has plenty of product in it. Apply mousse while it's wet, and then add in either dry shampoo or hairspray beforehand to make your hair easier to braid and to help the style hold well.

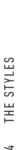

HIDDEN
paradise

*Looking for an awe-inspiring, unique braid that will make you the center of attention? This detailed style is made up of a **continuous fishtail braid, with large, twisted pieces** added to it from the front of the hairline that add an aura of mystery.*

difficulty
challenging

minimum hair length
shoulder blades

what you'll need
brush or comb
clear small elastic (or a color that matches your hair)

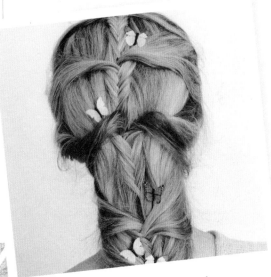

accessorize it!
Place butterfly clips randomly through the braid for a dash of whimsy.

1 Take a small section of hair from the center of your forehead. Use it to make a fishtail braid about 1 inch (2.5cm) long, pancaking as you go.

If you have bangs, take a section from just behind them

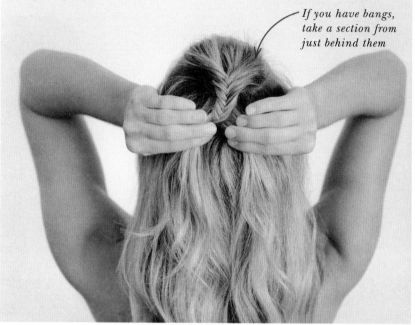

2 On one side of your head, twist a section of hair from the front of your hairline upward a couple times and add it into the braid.

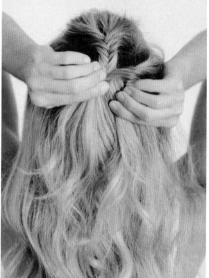

3 On the other side, twist a section of hair from the front of your hairline upward a couple times and add it into the braid.

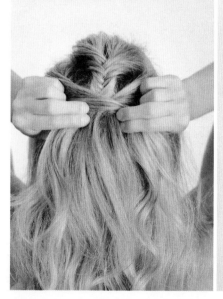

4 Fishtail braid without adding in any hair for about 1 or 2 inches (2.5 or 5cm).

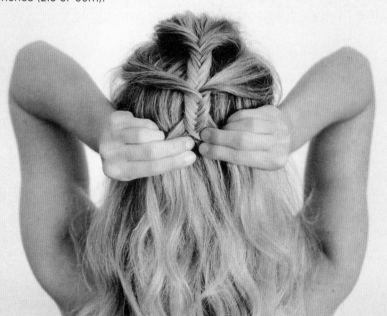

5 Repeat steps 2 through 4 until you reach the nape of the neck.

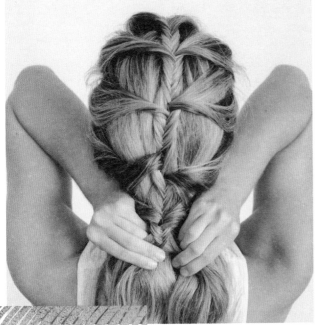

6 Fishtail braid to the ends of your hair. Secure the braid with an elastic.

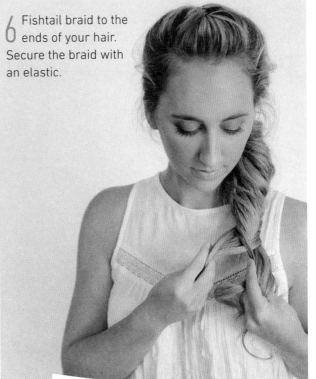

FINISHED LOOK

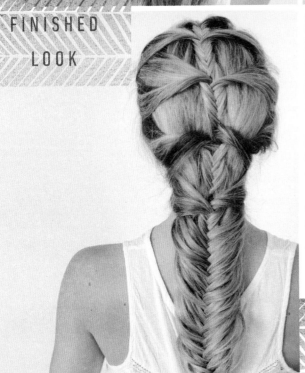

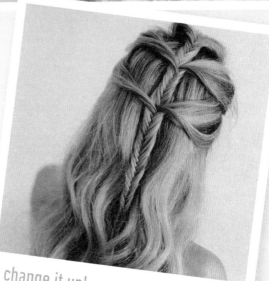

change it up!

After step 4, make this a half-updo by not adding anymore twists to the fishtail—simply braid it to the end.

ELF
maiden

*Are you a fantasy buff? Capture the same whimsy and wonder with this **easily done elfin style.** Expect a lot of oohs and ahhs at fairs and festivals from people impressed by your perfect, genre-appropriate look.*

difficulty
easy

minimum hair length
mid-back

what you'll need
comb
hair clip
bobby pins
clear small elastics (or a color that matches your hair)
hairspray

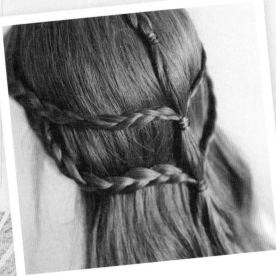

accessorize it!
Cover the elastics with small cuffs to give your style a more polished appearance.

This braid would look
great with some texture. If you
have naturally wavy hair, take
advantage of this by applying mousse
while your hair is still wet and drying your
hair with a diffuser attached to the dryer.
Dry on a low setting and hold your
head upside-down to get
maximum volume.

1 Part a section about 1 inch (2.5cm) wide, and then clip it. Pull the rest of your hair into a ponytail so it's out of the way.

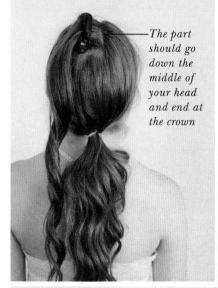

The part should go down the middle of your head and end at the crown

2 Dutch braid the 1-inch (2.5cm) section of hair. Braid about 2 inches (5cm) past when you stop adding in hair and secure with an elastic.

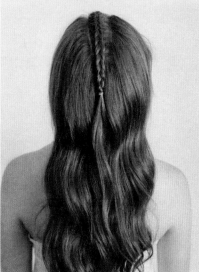

3 Take out the ponytail. Separate a section of hair on each side of your head, under the previous section you braided.

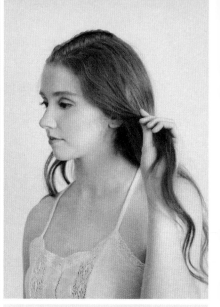

4 Basic braid a section to the end without adding in any hair. Bobby pin the end.

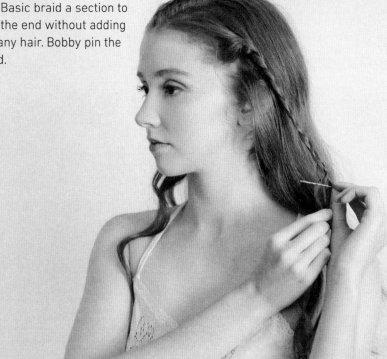

5 Repeat steps 3 and 4 on the other side.

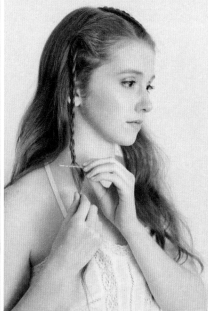

6 Leaving an unbraided 2-inch (5cm) tail on the Dutch braid finished in step 2, join the two braids with it in the back and secure with an elastic.

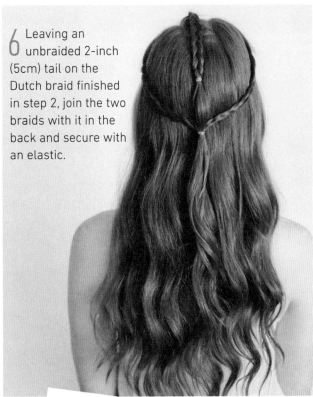

7 Repeat steps 3 through 6 to create a second row of braids. Finish the style with hairspray.

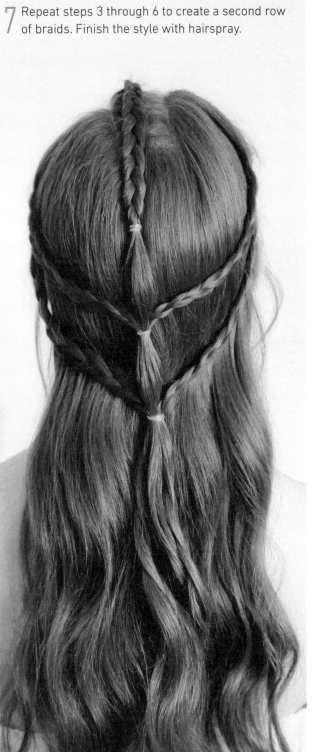

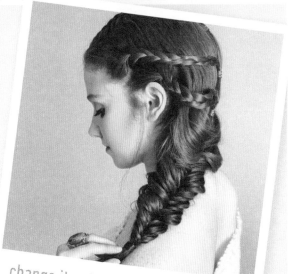

change it up!
Follow the instructions for steps 1 to 7, but fishtail the rest of the hair into a single braid.

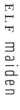

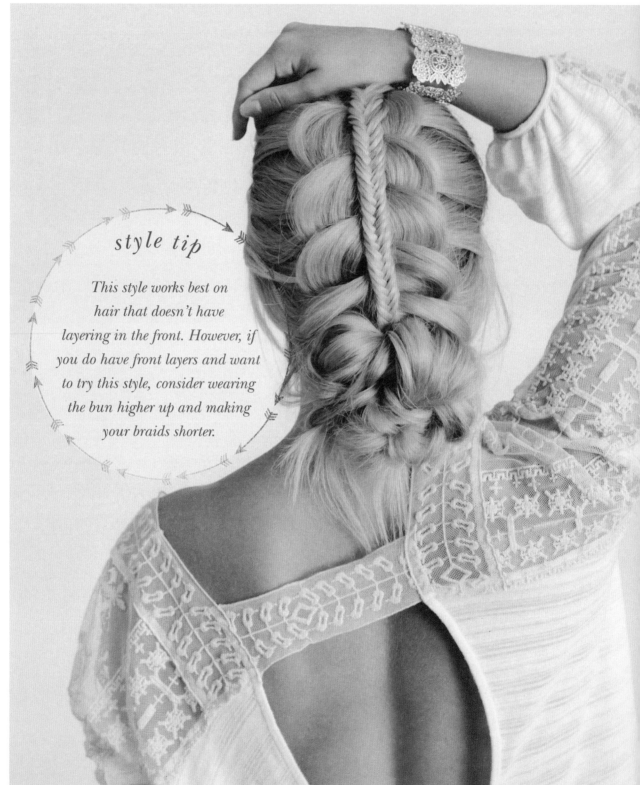

style tip

This style works best on hair that doesn't have layering in the front. However, if you do have front layers and want to try this style, consider wearing the bun higher up and making your braids shorter.

LINE IN THE
sand

difficulty
intermediate

minimum hair length
shoulder blades

what you'll need
hair clips
clear small elastics (or a color that matches your hair)
bobby pins
hairspray

*Make your hair a work of art— without much work! This style combines a **fishtail "line"** and a **widely pancaked Dutch braid** with a **low, messy bun** to create a beautifully layered look. Keep any accessories simple so you maintain people's focus on the unique design.*

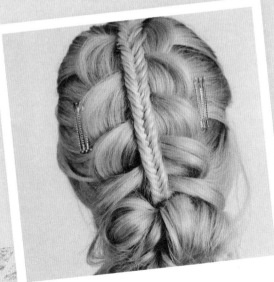

accessorize it!
Place a few decorative bobby pins right next to each other on either side of the Dutch braid to really show off the symmetry of the style.

1 Section out the fringe area and clip it away for later.

Optional: leave out wispy pieces in the front

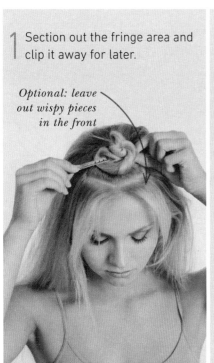

2 Dutch braid the remaining hair down the middle of the back of your head, leaving at least 6 inches (15.25cm) of tail unbraided. Secure with an elastic.

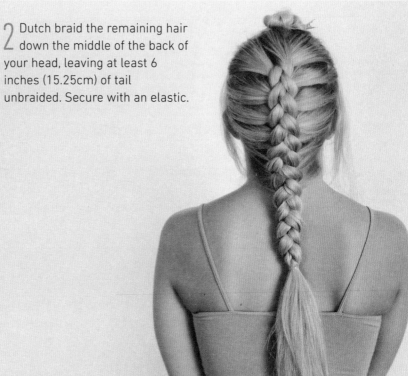

3 Pancake the Dutch braid as wide as you can make it without compromising the braid.

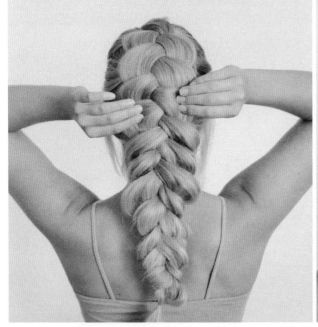

4 Unclip the fringe area and create a fishtail braid. Secure with an elastic.

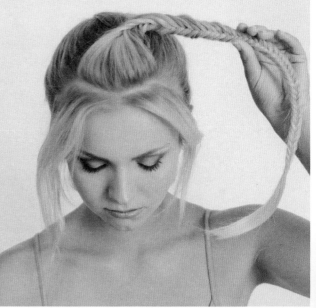

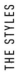

5 Place the fishtail braid directly down the middle and on top of the Dutch braid. Connect the two braids with bobby pins.

Slide the unopened bobby pins through and parallel to the braids

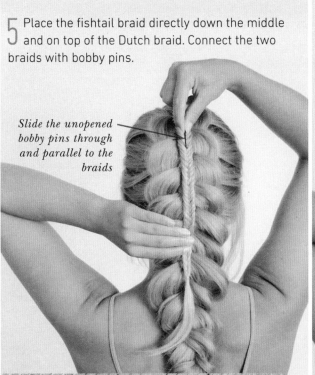

6 Wrap the tail of the Dutch braid to create a bun. Secure by sliding in bobby pins from the perimeter of the bun to the hair at your scalp. Finish the style with hairspray.

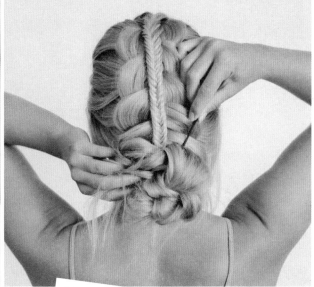

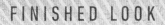

FINISHED LOOK

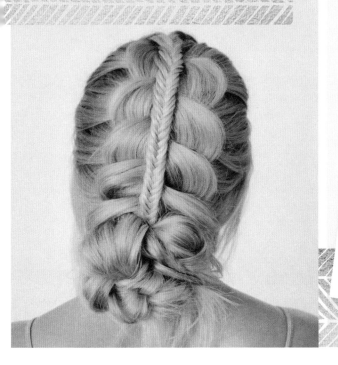

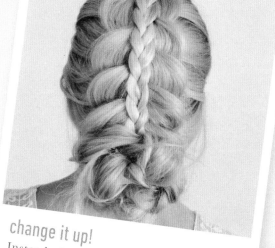

change it up!
Instead of a fishtail, try pairing the Dutch braid with a basic braid.

pure
INNOCENCE

If you want to tap into your sweeter, more innocent bohemian side, this **twisted side braid** *is for you. It's also a great option if you're in the middle of growing out your bangs, because your hair will be pulled back away from your face.*

difficulty
easy

minimum hair length
shoulder blades

what you'll need
bobby pins

clear small elastics (or a color that matches your hair)

hairspray

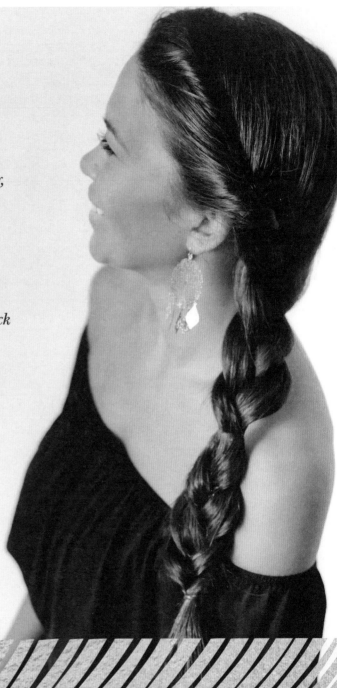

1 Begin twisting your fringe area away from your face.

2 Continue picking up hair from your hairline and adding it to the twist.

3 Secure the twist with bobby pins by sliding them upward into the twist.

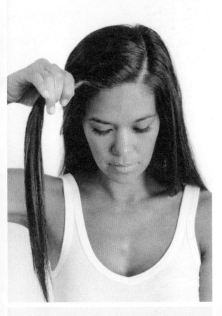
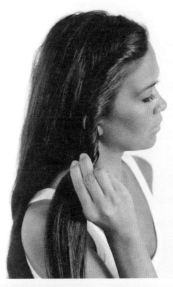
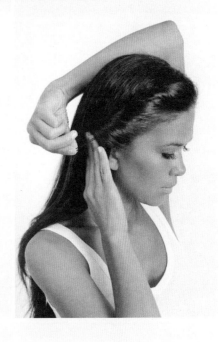

4 Divide the remaining hair into three sections and create a basic braid halfway down. Secure the middle with an elastic.

5 Create a basic braid with the remaining hair. Secure the end with an elastic band. Finish the style with hairspray.

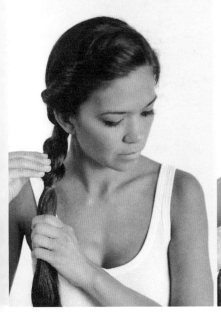

style tip

If you're having trouble with twisting your fringe, try curling the front of your hair away from your face to help encourage the hair to go in the direction of the twist.

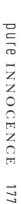

BOHO
ingénue

Add a splash of romance to your hair with this **elegant faux braid.** Despite its beautifully woven appearance, it requires no braiding skills at all, making it an **excellent beginner style.** Plus, it stays in well, giving you another reason to add it to your styling arsenal.

minimum hair length
mid-back

what you'll need
rat tail comb
clear ponytail elastics (or a color that matches your hair)
clear small elastics (or a color that matches your hair)
bobby pins
hairspray

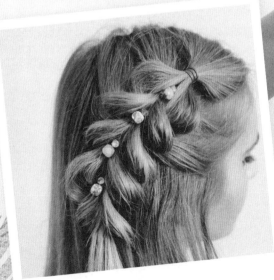

accessorize it!
To add some playfulness to the style, slide sparkle-tipped bobby pins upward into each elastic.

The trick to this style is to
include a lot of hair in each
section. If you begin with sections
that are too small, your braid will look
a lot less full and voluminous, and the
elastics will show. A trick to help you
avoid such trouble is to try starting
farther back on your head.

1 Part your hair to one side. On the heavy side of the part, section out a piece of hair in the front using a rat tail comb. Secure with an elastic near the top.

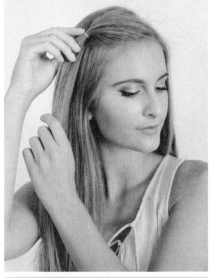

2 Pin the first ponytail out of the way. Make a second ponytail under the first, a little more toward the back of your head.

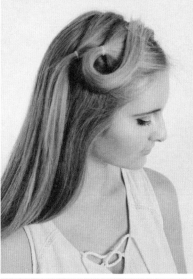

3 Unpin the first ponytail and split it into two equal sections.

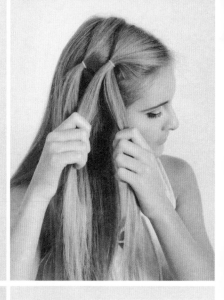

4 Place each half of the first ponytail on either side of the second. Join the two halves back together underneath it.

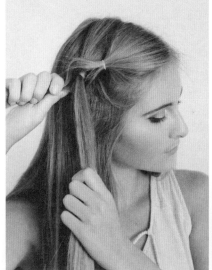

5 Secure the halves with an elastic and pancake them.

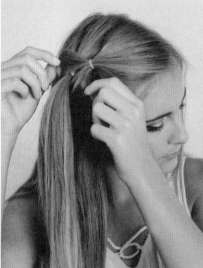

6 Make a third ponytail underneath the second one. This one should, as before, be a little more toward the back of your head.

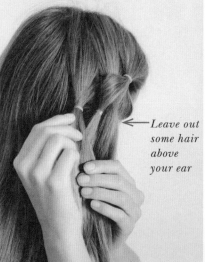

Leave out some hair above your ear

7 Split the second ponytail in half. Bring it around the section you joined in step 5, join it with the third ponytail, and secure with an elastic.

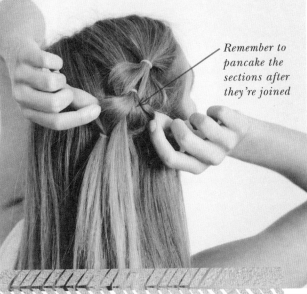

Remember to pancake the sections after they're joined

8 Repeat steps 3 through 5 with the two remaining sections, without making any new ponytails, until you run out of hair. Gently pancake each section a little more if desired. Finish the style with hairspray.

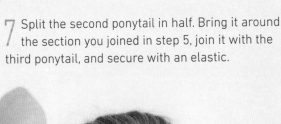

FINISHED LOOK

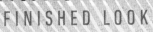

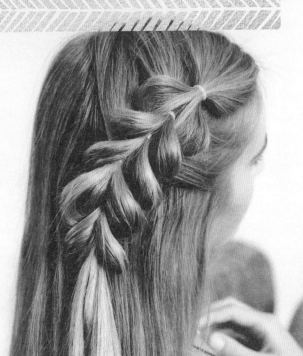

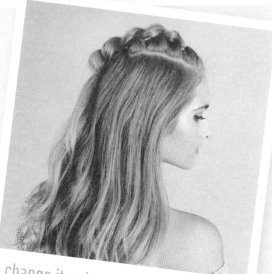

change it up!

Give this style a punk-rock feel by making your sections in the middle of the head to simulate a mohawk parting!

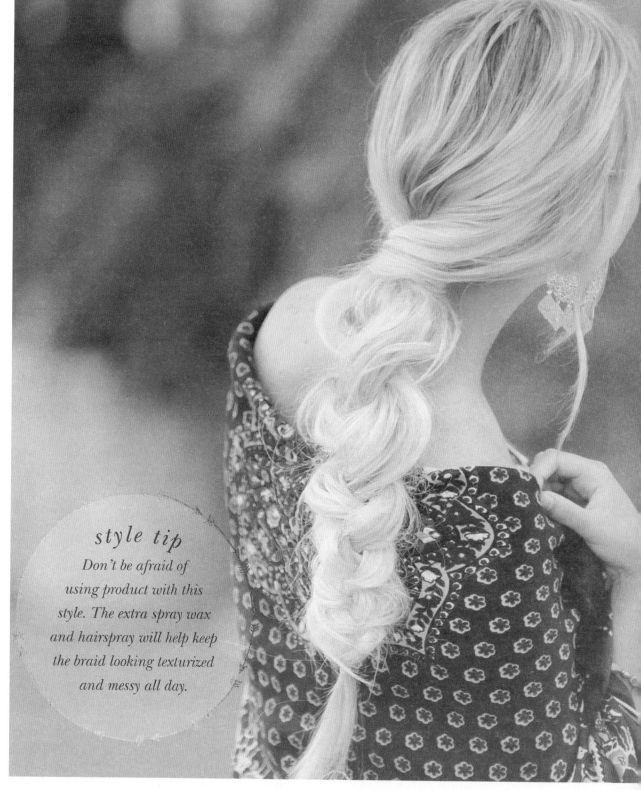

style tip

Don't be afraid of
using product with this
style. The extra spray wax
and hairspray will help keep
the braid looking texturized
and messy all day.

CATWALK
chic

difficulty
easy

minimum hair length
mid-back

what you'll need
hair clips
clear ponytail elastic (or a color that matches your hair)
spray wax
bobby pins
clear small elastic (or a color that matches your hair)
hairspray

Sometimes a simple **deconstructed braid** is all you need to spice up your normal hair routine. Whether you wear it casual or formal, this **ultra-textured braid** will make you look like you've just stepped off the runway.

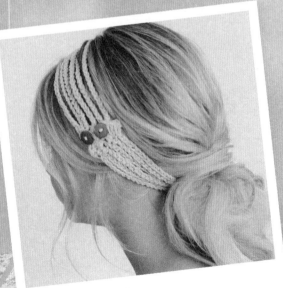

accessorize it!
A casual crocheted headband with six strands gives the style a Grecian look. Note how the button accents are left showing, to add a bit of visual interest.

1 Separate your hair into one large section in the back and two smaller sections on the sides. Clip them away.

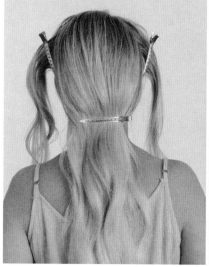

2 Pull the large back section into a very low ponytail and secure with an elastic. Spray the entire ponytail with spray wax.

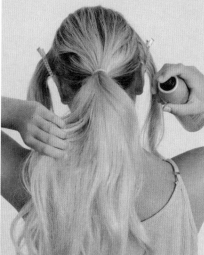

3 Take the right side section, cross it over the elastic band, and wrap it repeatedly around the elastic until it's entirely wound. Secure with a bobby pin.

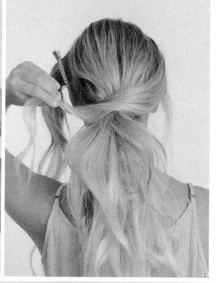

4 Take the left side section, cross it over the elastic band, and wrap it around the elastic until it's almost completely around it. Secure with a bobby pin.

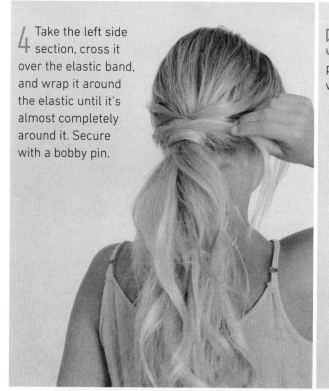

5 Create a loose basic braid with the ponytail and secure with an elastic.

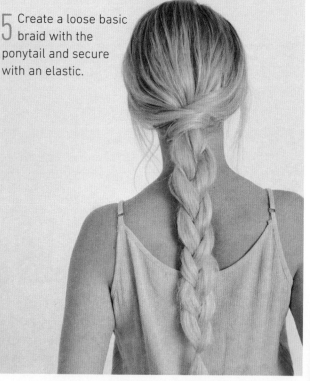

6 Pancake the braid and rub the loops between your fingers to create texture. Finish the style with hairspray.

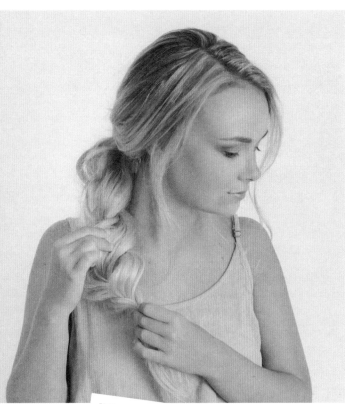

style tip

Rubbing the loops in step 6 is meant to get the hair frizzy. Just hold each loop lightly between your thumb and index finger and rub your fingertips together a few times, as if you're making the Italian gesture for "money."

FINISHED LOOK

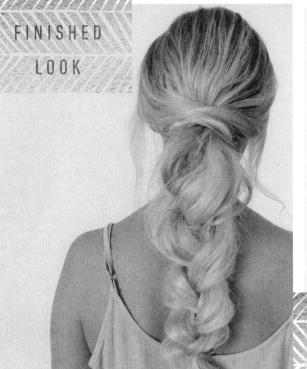

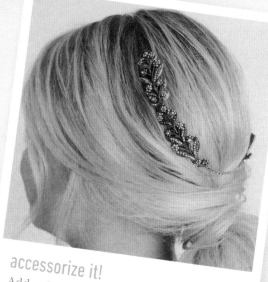

accessorize it!

Add a delicate headband to the top of your hair to take this hairstyle from simple to spectacular.

WILD
CHILD

*A **messy mini-Dutch mohawk** is just the beginning of this impressive **half-up style**. This ultra-bohemian look will make you stand out in a crowd, so wear it with a sassy attitude when going out on the town or singing along at a concert.*

difficulty
intermediate

minimum hair length
shoulder blades

what you'll need
large-barrel (1½ in.; 35mm) curling wand or iron
hair clip
clear ponytail elastics (or a color that matches your hair)
clear small elastics (or a color that matches your hair)
teasing comb
hairspray

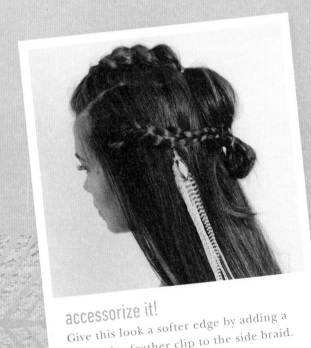

accessorize it!
Give this look a softer edge by adding a decorative feather clip to the side braid.

1 Create beach waves. Section out the mohawk area on top of your head. Clip away the rest of your hair.

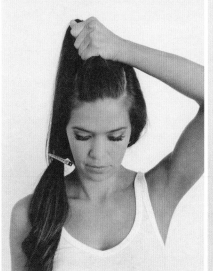

2 Create a Dutch braid with the mohawk section, finishing at the crown of your head. Secure the end with an elastic.

Leave the hair below the elastic unbraided

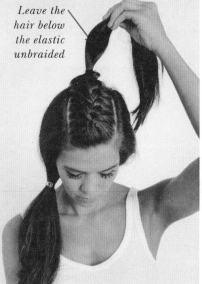

3 Unclip the right-front side of your hair and use it to create a basic braid.

Leave out hair around your face

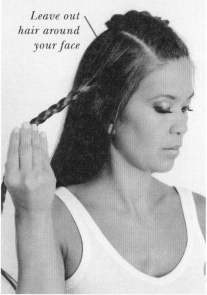

4 Repeat step 3 with hair from the left-front side. Secure the ends of each braid with an elastic.

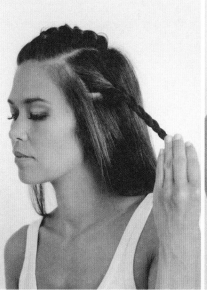

5 Unclip the rest of your hair and allow it to hang loose. Tease the underside of the hair hanging down from the mohawk section.

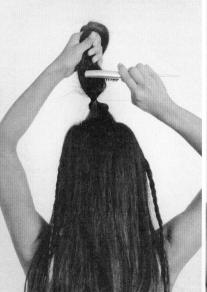

6 Join the two side braids together in the back, adding in hair from the ponytail section of the mohawk.

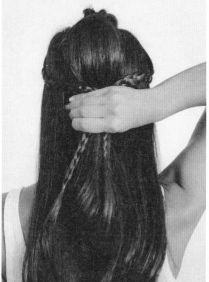

7 Start to place the three sections into a ponytail, but don't pull the hair all the way through the elastic. This creates a half-bun.

8 Pancake the Dutch braid by pulling on the loops.

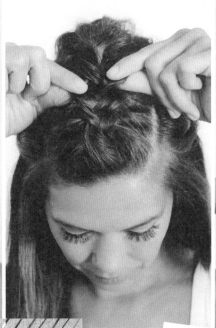

9 Gently pull on the hair at the crown for volume while holding onto the half-bun. Finish the style with hairspray.

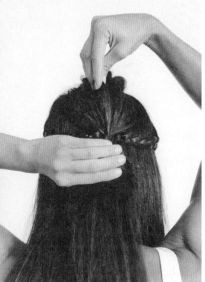

FINISHED LOOK

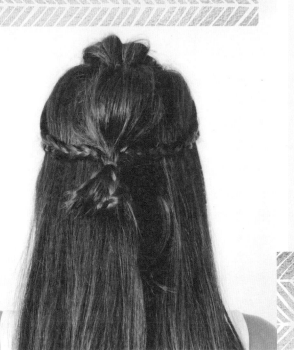

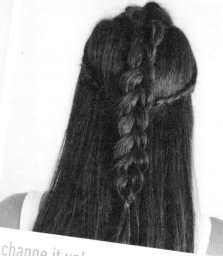

change it up!

Connect the two side braids in the back, and then finish the mohawk with a basic braid to lay over top.

ABOUT THE AUTHORS

HEIDI MARIE GARRETT is a licensed hair and makeup artist specializing in weddings and formal events, as well as a certified cosmetology educator trained to teach various skills to fellow beauty industry professionals. Although she grew up playing soccer and football, Heidi knew from a very young age that she would be a hairstylist and, after graduating from college with a Bachelor's degree in business, she began pursuing her passion. She has had the opportunity to travel domestically and internationally for clients. From 2013 to 2015, she volunteered in Cambodia on multiple occasions and taught local women the art and science of hairdressing, as well as life skills. What Heidi loves most about her job is the opportunity to connect with strangers and help them discover their potential, either in regard to their own natural beauty or their skills as a stylist. Heidi and her husband, Joshua, reside in Southern California.

KATIE ROSSI is a cosmetologist of 10 years. Her interest in braiding started when her oldest daughter, Abella, began preschool. Beginning on the first day of school, Katie braided Abella's hair into a different style each day. She was determined never to repeat the same style twice. Soon, people around the school began commenting that they always looked forward to seeing what she would come up with each day. This inspired Katie to start documenting each braid on social media, and it unexpectedly exploded into an account with tons of enthusiastic followers, asking her to show them how the styles were done. Katie's greatest passion is teaching people how to braid, and inspiring people of all ages to find their creative side and to learn as much as they can from every avenue possible. Katie lives in Arroyo Grande, California.

ACKNOWLEDGMENTS

HEIDI MARIE GARRETT:

This book has allowed me to come full circle in many aspects of my career and my life. I want to thank the editors, art directors, publishing company, my co-author, the models, and all the rest who have contributed to this book for allowing me to be a part of its creation alongside you. I will forever be grateful for the friend who encouraged me to start doing hair tutorials in my bathroom all those years ago. Thank you to my mom and dad and all of my family and friends who have helped grow my passion since its infancy in ways they probably don't realize. To my husband—who knows my heart, and who lets me be my wild self and do what I love while keeping me spiritually sound—I love you.

KATIE ROSSI:

I would first like to thank the amazing team of women who helped put this book together and made it all happen: my co-author, Heidi, who is such an inspiration to me; editors Nathalie Mornu and Kayla Dugger; art director and designer Becky Batchelor; and photographer Katherine Scheele. I also appreciate all of the gorgeous models who I had the pleasure of working with. I want to thank my husband, Ryan, who makes what I do possible and who gave me my two beautiful children. Thanks as well to Jan, my mom, my rock, my teacher, and my best friend. I thank my dad, Douglas, and sister, Heather, who share my love of photography and have helped me grow tremendously. I also give thanks to my grandma, Nancy, who passed down her creative genes to me. And, of course, a big thanks to my beautiful daughters, Abella and Charlie, who have sat through endless hours of braiding so that I could follow my passion and share it with the world.

FROM THE PUBLISHER:

The publisher is grateful to Lexy and Katherine Scheele for wardrobe assistance, and also wishes to thank the models whose gorgeous locks grace these pages: Alexandra Elliott, Amanda Matthews, Amanda Naaman, Victoria Olson, Josie Sanders, Lexy Scheele, Christina Taylor, and Rachel Wood. A special thanks goes to Josie Sanders for her help in naming the hairstyles.

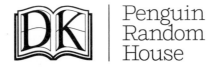

Publisher: Mike Sanders

Associate Publisher: Billy Fields

Acquisitions Editor: Nathalie Mornu

Development Editor: Kayla Dugger

Cover and Book Designer: Rebecca Batchelor

Photographer: Katherine Scheele

Prepress: Brian Massey

Proofreader: Jamie Fields

First American Edition, 2017
Published in the United States by DK Publishing
6081 E. 82nd Street, Indianapolis, Indiana 46250

Copyright © 2017 Dorling Kindersley Limited
A Penguin Random House Company
17 18 19 20   10 9 8 7 6 5 4 3 2 1
001–301844–March/2017

Published in the United States by Dorling Kindersley Limited.

ISBN: 978-1-4654-6037-0
Library of Congress Catalog Card Number: 2016950731

Note: This publication contains the opinions and ideas of its author(s). It is intended to provide helpful and informative material on the subject matter covered. It is sold with the understanding that the author(s) and publisher are not engaged in rendering professional services in the book. If the reader requires personal assistance or advice, a competent professional should be consulted. The author(s) and publisher specifically disclaim any responsibility for any liability, loss, or risk, personal or otherwise, which is incurred as a consequence, directly or indirectly, of the use and application of any of the contents of this book.

DK books are available at special discounts when purchased in bulk for sales promotions, premiums, fund-raising, or educational use. For details, contact: DK Publishing Special Markets, 345 Hudson Street, New York, New York 10014 or SpecialSales@dk.com.

Printed and bound in China

All images © Dorling Kindersley Limited
For further information see: www.dkimages.com

www.dk.com

A WORLD OF IDEAS:
SEE ALL THERE IS TO KNOW